# PRIMER OF EEG

# Primer of EEG
## With a Mini-Atlas

### A. James Rowan, M.D.
*Professor of Neurology, Mount Sinai School of Medicine;*
*Director of Electroencephalography, Mount Sinai Hospital;*
*Chief, Neurology Service, Bronx VA Medical Center*

### Eugene Tolunsky, M.D.
*Mount Sinai Hospital, New York*

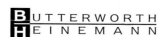

**BUTTERWORTH**
**HEINEMANN**

*An Imprint of Elsevier*

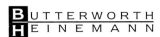

*An Imprint of Elsevier*

The Curtis Center
Independence Square West
Philadelphia, Pennsylvania 19106

**Library of Congress Cataloging-in-Publication Data**

A primer of EEG: with a mini-atlas / edited by A. James Rowan, Eugene Tolunsky.–1st ed.
    p. ; cm.
    Includes bibliographical references and index.

    ISBN-13: 978-0-7506-7476-8        ISBN-10: 0-7506-7476-8
    1. Electroencephalography. 2. Electroencephalography–Atlases. I. Rowan, A. J. II. Tolunsky, Eugene.
    [DNLM: 1. Electroencephalography–methods. 2. Electroencephalography–Atlases. WL 150 P953 2003]
    RC386.6.E43P737 2005
    616.8'047547–dc21                                                                    2003041823

*Acquisitions Editor:* Susan F. Pioli
*Development Editor:* Laurie Ancllo

Printed in the United States of America

ISBN-13: 978-0-7506-7476-8
ISBN-10: 0-7506-7476-8

Last digit is the print number: 9   8   7

# TABLE OF CONTENTS

# PREFACE

Neurology residents pursuing an elective in clinical neurophysiology often ask what textbooks they should consult or purchase. There are, of course, a number of excellent resources, some quite compendious. The resident physician, when confronted with detailed EEG textbooks, is a bit daunted at the prospect of delving into them. Because less and less time is devoted to EEG in the average residency, often a single month, the instructor faces a considerable challenge: how to impart as much knowledge as possible in a limited time. We felt that help was needed; that is, a teaching companion that would distill the essentials of EEG in an accessible format, allowing the resident to make the most of his or her limited time in the discipline.

This text is also intended for those pursuing a fellowship in clinical neurophysiology. Of course fellows have a less difficult task than residents as they have at least one and possibly two years to master the requisite skills. More time is available to consult the available textbooks and study the literature. Still, it is difficult at the outset to synthesize textbook learning and practical experience in interpretation. We believe this volume will provide fellows with a jump-start toward their goal of becoming expert electroencephalographers. In addition to trainees, this book should appeal to other physicians who order studies in circumstances particular to their specialties. Internists, psychiatrists, critical care physicians, and ICU specialists come to mind. Each of these encounter patients with potential CNS involvement such as altered mental status, possible seizures, and toxic-metabolic disorders. In addition, attending neurologists not specializing in EEG may find the book useful for brushing up on essentials. Finally, we hope the work will appeal to EEG technicians, both for its technical and clinical discussions.

The reader will be taken through a broad sweep of clinical EEG, touching on topics such as the value of the test, normal and abnormal findings, specific disease entities, pitfalls to avoid, and how to approach the task of interpretation. Because of the important and often underappreciated role of the EEG in diagnosis and treatment of status epilepticus, we discuss this topic in some detail including clinical characteristics, the wide variety of electrographic findings, and tips on treatment under EEG control. We also include some thoughts on the use of EEG in guiding treatment of epilepsy as well as its role in determining prognosis.

To supplement these discussions the reader will find a Mini-Atlas of electrographic findings that we believe will bring many of the sometimes difficult-to-describe phenomena to life. The Atlas demonstrates examples of normal and abnormal records along with commonly encountered artifacts and normal variants. In-text cross-references to the Mini-Atlas are designated A-1, A-2, etc.

For this introductory text we decided to confine our discussion to the EEG in children and adults. Neonatal EEG is a highly specialized field that we felt was outside the scope of this work. We also have omitted topics such as evoked potentials, magnetoencephalography, electromyography, and intraoperative monitoring. These topics are explored in currently available textbooks, many of which are listed in the Appendix. This primer arose in the background of actual teaching sessions for the groups mentioned above. Thus, one will find throughout its pages a generous helping of practical experience. We hope that our readers will find the work convenient, of practical value, not too onerous to read, and even enjoyable in places.

A.J.R.

E.T.

# ACKNOWLEDGMENTS

The authors are grateful to R. Eugene Ramsay, MD, Dennis B. Smith, MD, and Donald F. Scott, MD for their invaluable guidance and detailed suggestions for improving the manuscript. We also tip our hats to our neurology residents for their support, in particular Alex Boro, MD, and Nilay Shah, MD, Steven Gunzler, MD and Kenneth Fox, MD for their assistance in helping to make the book user friendly. We acknowledge our EEG technologists, Nina Michaels, Yvonne Heyward, and Mary Ann Sostak, who provided the excellent recordings from which the Mini-Atlas of EEG was assembled. Finally, we are indebted to Susan Pioli, our publisher, who provided support and encouragement from the beginning.

# INTRODUCTION:
# THE UTILITY OF THE EEG

Since its earliest days, the EEG has been critical in the diagnosis and management of epilepsy. A wide variety of paroxysmal phenomena are associated with particular types of seizure disorders. Thus, the EEG not only provides support for the diagnosis but also is instrumental in epilepsy classification. Further, patients with epilepsy are often followed with serial recordings. New epileptiform findings may be discovered in those with increasing seizure frequency. Other pathology may be suggested by discovery of a new EEG abnormality. A lessening of epileptiform activity may suggest improvement of the patient's condition, although this is not consistent. Of equal importance, if not more so, is the more recent development of prolonged EEG-video recording (24 hours or more) that allows simultaneous recording of a patient's clinical seizures and the associated electrographic abnormality. Detailed analysis of the clinical and associated electrographic phenomena is thus possible.

The EEG also has a primary role to play in the diagnosis and treatment of status epilepticus, a role that we believe is underappreciated. This applies not only to obvious repeated major seizures but also to another type of status, characterized by confusion or depression of consciousness. In these cases the EEG is the only test that confirms the diagnosis. We will discuss these topics in some depth.

Since Berger described changes in the EEG associated with epilepsy over 70 years ago, many additional uses of the EEG have been discovered. In fact, before the advent of imaging the EEG was the principal tool for investigating patients with cerebral disease – always preceding more invasive procedures such as arteriography and pneumoencephalography. Indeed, the arrival of computed tomography (CT), and later magnetic resonance imaging (MRI), resulted in gloom among electroencephalographers. It was felt that the use of EEG would wither in the face of this new competition. But news of its demise was premature. Thanks to the expansion of technology as well as more sophisticated applications of the test to various disease states, the EEG continues to occupy a strong position in the evaluation of neurological disease.

The EEG is useful in the investigation of neurological disorders other than epilepsy. For example, a common reason for ordering an EEG – especially by non-neurologists – is change in mental status. This non-specific diagnosis, with exceptions, is often best investigated by EEG, not imaging. Of course, both are usually required. Was the change in mental status secondary to: syncope? seizures? non-convulsive status epilepticus? metabolic causes? effects of medications? In these and other instances the study may reveal findings that point to the proper diagnosis. Each of these topics will be explored.

The EEG finds a role in the investigation of possible toxic-metabolic disorders. Although laboratory findings usually leads to the diagnosis, this is not always the case. The EEG provides clues that may support the presumed diagnosis, sometimes reveals surprising findings, and is often used to follow the patient's progress. Triphasic waves, for example, may point to hepatic encephalopathy. A marked excess of beta activity may suggest an overdose of barbiturates or benzodiazepines. Disruption of background rhythms with diffuse slowing is a common finding and suggests a non-focal process, possibly metabolic, in patients with changes in mental status.

Other important areas in which the EEG provides useful information are stroke, increased intracranial pressure, subdural collections, dementias and coma to name a few. The reader is referred to separate sections dealing with these issues.

We emphasize that a careful history will augment the diagnostic power of the electrographic findings. Note that the correlation of the history with the electrographic findings increases the EEG's utility. Not only should the clinician provide important historical details but a well-trained technician can supplement information on the request form by questioning the patient or consulting the accompanying chart.

In short, the EEG provides supplementary and often crucial information in a wide variety of neurological disorders. It is the goal of this book to awaken not only an appreciation of the test's diagnostic power but also an understanding of the many elements that lead to accurate EEG interpretation.

# 1

# ORIGIN AND TECHNICAL ASPECTS OF THE EEG

## ORIGIN OF THE EEG

The EEG records electrical activity from the cerebral cortex. Inasmuch as electrocortical activity is measured in microvolts ($\mu$V), it must be amplified by a factor of 1,000,000 in order to be displayed on a computer screen or in a write-out. Most of what we record is felt to originate from neurons, and there are a number of possible sources including action potentials, post-synaptic potentials, and chronic neuronal depolarization. Action potentials induce a brief (10 ms or less) local current in the axon with a very limited potential field. This makes them unlikely candidates. Post-synaptic potentials (PSPs) are considerably longer (50–200 ms), have a much greater field, and thus are more likely to be the primary generators of the EEG. Long-term depolarization of the neuron or even the glia could also play a role and produce EEG changes that would be recorded from an injured brain.

In the normal brain an action potential travels down the axon to the nerve terminal where a neurotransmitter is released. At the post-synaptic membrane the neurotransmitter produces a change in membrane conductance and trans-membrane potential. If the signal has an excitatory effect on the neuron it leads to a local reduction of the transmembrane potential (depolarization) and is called an excitatory post-synaptic potential (EPSP), typically located in the dendrites. If the signal has an inhibitory effect on the neuron it leads to local hyperpolarization and is called an inhibitory post-synaptic potential (IPSP), typically located on the cell body of the neuron. The combination of EPSPs and IPSPs induces currents that flow within and around the neuron with a potential field sufficient to be recorded on the scalp. It turns out that the typical duration of a PSP, 100 ms, is similar to the duration of the average alpha wave. The alpha rhythm, consisting of sinusoidal or rhythmic alpha waves, is the basic rhythmic frequency of the normal adult brain.

It is easy to understand how complex neuronal electrical activity generates irregular EEG signals that translate into seemingly random and ever-changing

EEG waves. Less obvious is the physiological explanation of the rhythmic character of certain EEG patterns seen both in sleep and wakefulness. The mechanisms underlying EEG rhythmicity, although not completely understood, are mediated through two main processes. The first is the interaction between cortex and thalamus. The activity of thalamic pacemaker cells leads to rhythmic cortical activation. For example, the cells in the nucleus reticularis of the thalamus have the pacing properties responsible for the generation of sleep spindles. The second is based on the functional properties of large neuronal networks in the cortex that have an intrinsic capacity for rhythmicity. The result of both mechanisms is the creation of recognizable EEG patterns, varying in different areas of neocortex, that allow us to make sense of the complex world of brain waves.

## TECHNICAL CONSIDERATIONS

The reader may find the following sections quite difficult at this early stage. The authors suggest that mastery of the technical details of the EEG will come with time. Perhaps it is best to peruse the discussion, noting its content and scope, and then go on to Chapter 2, the Normal EEG. Repeated reference to the technical discussions, combined with practical experience in interpreting the tracings, will ultimately result in a clear understanding of EEG fundamentals. Do not be discouraged!

The major problem in electroencephalography is the amplification of tiny currents 1,000,000 times, transducing the amplified potentials into a graphic representation that can be interpreted. Of course extracerebral potentials are likewise amplified (movements and the like), and these are many times the amplitude of electrocortical potentials. Thus, unless understood and corrected for, such interference or artifacts would obscure the underlying EEG. The electroencephalographer is quite different from the archeologist who spends a lifetime searching for artifacts. We try to obtain recordings that are artifact-free or, if artifacts are present, to exclude these from consideration and teach our students likewise. This presents considerable difficulties. Later, we will discuss artifacts in detail and illustrate clearly their many guises. At this point we will consider the technical factors that are indispensable in obtaining an artifact-free and thus interpretable record.

### Electrodes

Electrodes are simply the means by which the electrocortical potentials are conducted to the amplification apparatus. Essentially, standard EEG electrodes are small, non-reactive metal discs or cups applied to the scalp with a conductive paste. Several types of metals are used including gold, silver/silver chloride, tin, and platinum. Electrode contact must be firm in order to ensure low impedance (resistance to current flow), thus minimizing both electrode and environmental artifacts. For longer-term monitoring, especially if the patient is mobile, cup electrodes are affixed with collodion (a sort of glue), and a conductive gel is inserted between electrode and scalp through a small hole in the electrode itself. This procedure maintains recording integrity over prolonged periods.

Other types of electrodes are available but seldom used. Needle electrodes, formerly quite common, are not appropriate because of the risk of infection, discomfort, and poor recording quality. Nasopharyngeal electrodes were often used in patients suspected of harboring a temporal lobe paroxysmal abnormality. Today, they have fallen into disfavor due to their discomfort and susceptibility to a variety of artifacts. Some laboratories investigating patients for possible epilepsy surgery use sphenoidal electrodes, in addition to a standard scalp array, during routine recording and prolonged EEG-video monitoring. The electrode – a thin wire that is insulated except for the tip – is inserted through the mandibular notch via a hollow needle, the tip coming to rest near the foramen ovale. The needle is then removed, and the electrode remains in place. A spike originating in the deep temporal structures with limited surface representation may be well displayed at a sphenoidal electrode. We recommend that only an experienced operator should insert these electrodes.

**Electrode Placement**

Electrode placement is standardized in the United States and indeed in most other nations. This allows EEGs performed in one laboratory to be interpreted in another. The general problem is to record activity from various parts of the cerebral cortex in a logical, interpretable manner. Thanks to Dr. Herbert Jasper, a renowned electroencephalographer at the Montreal Neurological Institute, we have a logical, generally accepted system of electrode placement: the 10-20 International System of Electrode Placement. This system, which was developed during the 1950s, depends on accurate measurements of the skull, utilizing several distinctive landmarks. Essentially, a semicircumferential arc of the skull is taken in three planes – sagittal, coronal, and horizontal.

- The sagittal measurement extends from the nasion (the depression at the top of the nose) over the top of the head to the inion (the prominence in the midline at the base of the occiput). This defines the sagittal plane (Figure 1-1).

Now, three measurements are important in defining the other two planes. The first is one half (50%) the distance from the nasion to the inion, which becomes one marker of the vertex. The second and third are points above the nasion and inion, each 10 percent of the total sagittal measurement. These aid in establishing the horizontal plane.

- The coronal measurement extends from a point just anterior to the tragus (the cartilaginous protrusion at the front of the external ear), traversing the

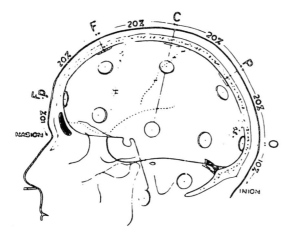

**Figure 1-1** Lateral view of the skull to show methods of measurement from nasion to inion at the mid-line. $F_p$ is frontal pole position, F is the frontal line of electrodes, C is the central line of electrodes, P is the parietal line of electrodes and 0 is the occipital line. Percentages indicate represent proportions of the measured distance from the nasion to the inion. Note that the central line is 50% of this distance. The frontal pole and occipital electrodes are 10% from the nasion and inion respectively. Twice this distance, or 20%, separates the outer line of electrodes. (Reprinted with permission from Jasper HH. Report of the committee on methods of clinical examination in electroencephalography. *Electroenceph Clin Neurophysiol* 1958;10:370–375.)

mid-point of the sagittal measurement, to the same point on the opposite side. This defines the coronal plane. The intersection of the halfway (50%) points of the sagittal and coronal measurements is the location of the vertex and thus the Cz electrode (Figure 1-2).

The point above the tragus on each side that is 10 percent of the total coronal measurement, along with the 10 percent points above the nasion and inion of the total sagittal measurement, will be used to define the horizontal measurement

- The horizontal measurement is taken separately on both sides of the head. It extends from a point above the inion that is 10 percent of the total sagittal measurement, through the point above the tragus that are 10 percent of the coronal measurement, to the point that is 10 percent above the inion. These measurements define the horizontal plane (Figure 1-3).

We are now ready to define the loci for electrode placement. Standard electrode designations follow (Figures 1-4–1-6). These should be memorized during the student's first day of his or her elective. (Note: by convention, electrodes designated with odd numbers are located on the left; those with even numbers on the right.)

Fp1/Fp2 = fronto-polar or prefrontal (on the forehead – records activity from the frontal poles)

F3/F4 = mid-frontal (over the frontal lobe – records frontal activity)

C3/C4 = central (roughly over the fissure of Rolando, also known as the central sulcus)

P3/P4 = parietal (records parietal activity)

O1/O2 = occipital (records occipital activity)

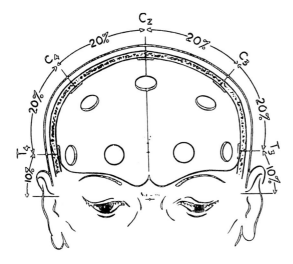

**Figure 1-2** Frontal view of the skull showing the method of measurement for the central line of electrodes as described in the text. (Reprinted with permission from Jasper HH. Report of the committee on methods of clinical examination in electroencephalography. *Electroenceph Clin Neurophysiol* 1958;10:370–375.)

F7/F8 = inferior frontal, sometimes called anterior temporal (records activity from the orbital frontal, lateral frontal, and anterior temporal regions)

T3/T4 = mid-temporal (records activity from the anterior and mid-temporal regions)

T5/T6 = posterior temporal (records activity from the posterior temporal regions)

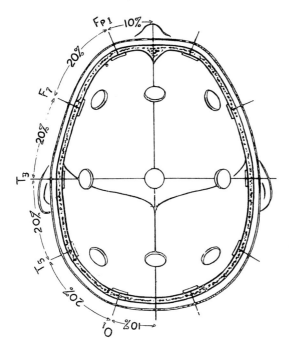

**Figure 1-3** Superior view with cross-section of skull through the temporal line of electrodes illustrating the 10–20 system applied in this direction and described in the text. (Reprinted with permission from Jasper HH. Report of the committee on methods of clinical examination in electroencephalography. *Electroenceph Clin Neurophysiol* 1958;10:370–375.)

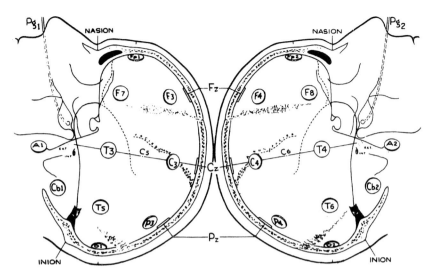

**Figure 1-4** The lateral view of left and right hemispheres showing all standard electrode positions, omitting intermediate positions (such as C5 and C6) which are used only for special studies with more closely spaced electrodes. These drawings were made from a series of X-ray projections with true lateral views. The location of principal fissures was determined by silver clips placed at operation and by other anatomical studies described in the text. The location of pharyngeal electrodes (Pg$_1$ and Pg$_2$) was also obtained from X-ray studies with these electrodes in place. (Reprinted with permission from Jasper HH. Report of the committee on methods of clinicalexamination in electroencephalography. *Electroenceph Clin Neurophysiol* 1958;10: 370–375.)

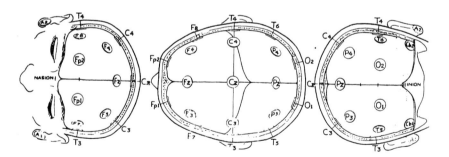

**Figure 1-5** Frontal superior and posterior views showing all the standard electrode positions as described in the text. (Reprinted with permission from Jasper HH. Report of the committee on methods of clinical examination in electroencephalography. *Electroenceph Clin Neurophysiol* 1958;10:370–375.)

Fz, Cz, Pz = midline electrodes in the frontal, central and parietal regions (record potentials from the midline and the mesial surfaces of the hemispheres)

A1/A2 = ear referential electrodes (while used as references, they also record activity from the mid-temporal regions)

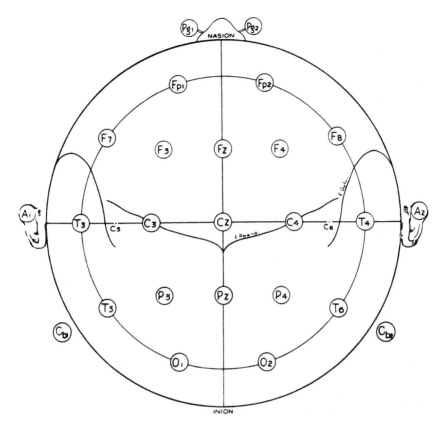

**Figure 1-6** A single plane projection of the head, showing all standard positions and the locations of rolandic and Sylvian fissures. The outer circle was drawn at the level of the nasion and inion. The inner circle represents the temporal line of electrodes. This diagram provides a useful stamp for the indication of electrode placements in routine recording. (Reprinted with permission from Jasper HH. Report of the committee on methods of clinical examination in electroencephalography. *Electroenceph Clin Neurophysiol* 1958;10:370–375.)

T1/T2 = so-called true anterior temporal electrodes (records activity from the anterior temporal regions). The electrode is located 1 cm above a point that is one-third the anterior distance on a line from the external auditory canal to the lateral canthus of the eye.

Sp1/Sp2 = sphenoidal electrodes (not part of the 10-20 system, but they record activity from the infero-mesial surface of the temporal lobes)

### How to Measure for Electrode Placement

First, measure the sagittal plane, noting the distance in centimeters from the nasion to the inion. With a red wax pencil, mark the point above the nasion that is 10 percent of the total measurement, and the point above the inion that also is

10 percent of the total. Divide and mark the remaining 80 percent into four segments, each 20 percent of the total measurement (thus, the 10-20 system). The first 20 percent point defines Fz, the second Cz and the third Pz – the midline electrodes (z = zero). The final 20 percent is the distance between Pz and your point 10 percent above the inion. Thus, the total is 100 percent (Figure 1-1).

Next, measure the coronal plane that extends from the point anterior to the tragus to the same point on the opposite side, making sure that your tape measure traverses the Cz point on the sagittal measurement.. The first 10 percent points define T3 and T4, the mid-temporal electrodes. The next 20 percent points then define C3 and C4, the central electrodes. The remaining 20 percent segments represent the distance from C3 and C4 to Cz (Figure 1-2).

Now, measure the horizontal plane. The tape measure should be placed between the 10 percent points of the sagittal measurement, extending through the T3 on the left and T4 on the right. The 10 percent points of the horizontal plane define Fp1 and Fp2 anteriorly (the fronto-polar electrodes), and O1 and O2 posteriorly (the occipital electrodes). The 20 percent points define F7 and F8 anteriorly (the inferior frontal electrodes) and T5 and T6 posteriorly (the posterior temporal electrodes). The remaining two 20 percent segments represent the distances between F7 and T3, and T3 and T5 on the left, and between F8 and T4, and T4 and T6 on the right. (Remember, the locations of T3 and T4 have already been established during measurement of the coronal plane (Figure 1-3).)

Finally, F3 and F4 are defined by the halfway points between F7 and Fz on the left, and F8 and Fz on the right. Similarly, P3 and P4 are defined by the halfway points between T5 and Pz on the left, and T6 and Pz on the right.

An observation: the 10-20 system is not the only system of electrode placement. It does have its problems. For example, the F7 and F8 electrodes are probably placed too high for optimal definition of anterior temporal activity [some laboratories routinely use T1 and T2 (so-called true anterior temporal electrodes)]. Likewise, the T5 and T6 electrodes are too high for good definition of posterior temporal activity (electrodes placed interior to T5 and T6 are sometimes used). Nonetheless, the system is serviceable and generally accepted for routine EEG recording.

While the 10-20 system may sound a bit complicated, in practice it is quite easily carried out. Nonetheless, there is nothing like actually measuring and placing the electrodes yourself under the guidance of an experienced EEG technologist. We recommend that all residents perform at least two to three supervised EEGs during their EEG rotations. Fellows should do more until they are confident of their ability measure accurately and apply electrodes properly.

## Potential Fields

Before discussing how we display the electrical information recorded by the electrodes, the reader should understand the concept of the potential field. The summation of IPSPs and EPSPs in a neuronal net creates electrical currents that flow in and around the cells. The flow of current creates a field that spreads out from the origin of an electrical event (such as a spike or slow wave), much the same as the concentric rings created on a glassy pond when one tosses a pebble onto its surface. Potential fields are usually oval in shape and may be quite restricted or very widespread. The field's effect diminishes as the distance from the source increases. This means that events producing maximal voltage on a particular electrode will affect adjacent electrodes as well, but to a lesser extent as the potential wanes from the point of origin (Figure 1-7).

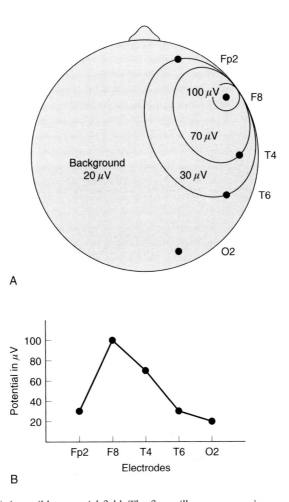

**Figure 1-7** (A) A possible potential field. The figure illustrates a maximum negative potential of 100 μV at F8. The field spreads to involve T4 at a lower potential of 70 μV, and then to Fp2 and T6 at 30 μV. The background unaffected by the potential averages 20 μV. (B) Another way to depict the same data. Note the steep rise from Fp2 to F8, declining successively to T4 and T6. O2 has the same potential as the rest of the background.

## Amplification

Easiest to understand is the simple amplifier. Input from a single active electrode is conducted to the amplifier and compared to ground (earth). Thus, the output consists of the potential difference between the active electrode and ground. Electrocortical potentials as well as other environmental potentials affecting the electrode (e.g. 60 Hz interference) are displayed in the output. In differential amplification signals from two active leads are conducted to the amplifier, thus measuring the potential difference between the two. In this case, any signal that affects both inputs identically (say 60 Hz) will result in no potential difference and thus will not be displayed or be much reduced. This phenomenon is termed in-phase cancellation (Figure 1-8).

We are now in a position to consider methods of recording electrocortical potentials so that we can make sense of them. Recalling that amplifiers record potential difference between two incoming signals, we can record the potential difference between two electrodes on the scalp (bipolar recording). On the other hand, we can record the potential difference between a scalp electrode and

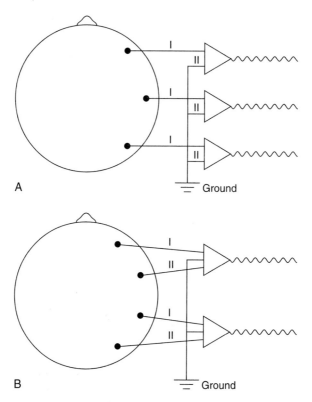

**Figure 1-8** (A) Simple amplifier. Input from each active electrode is compared with ground. (B) Differential amplifier. Here, potential difference is measured between two active electrodes.

another point (the reference) that, ideally, is unaffected by cerebral potentials or other interference (referential recording). Unfortunately it is virtually impossible to achieve this ideal, but certain references (e.g. the ears) are quite serviceable. These two types of recording, along with their advantages and disadvantages, are discussed below.

## Bipolar Recording

Bipolar recording electronically links successive electrodes (known as a chain or line), the voltage at one electrode being compared to the voltage affecting adjacent electrodes (potential difference). Take for example the chain of electrodes on the right side starting at Fp2 and ending with O2 (known as the temporal chain: Fp2→F8 →T4 →T6 → O2). The voltage of an event (e.g. a spike) occurring at F8 is compared with the potential field of the event that affects adjacent electrodes, in this case Fp2 and T4. The voltage at T4 is compared with the voltages at F8 and T6, and so on. The voltage comparisons take place by conducting the signal recorded by a particular electrode to opposite sides of two adjacent amplifiers (for example Input II in the first and Input I in the second), each amplifying the signal equally but with opposite deflections on the display or write-out.

Now: one additional bit of information is needed in order to interpret bipolar recording.

Remember: each amplifier has two inputs, I and II. (Some still use the term Grid, recalling the early era of vacuum tubes. In the United Kingdom, the terms black and white leads are used.) By convention, the rule for understanding the display or write-out is:

IF INPUT I BECOMES NEGATIVE WITH RESPECT TO INPUT II, THERE IS AN UPWARD DEFLECTION. (It follows, therefore, that the opposite situation is also true: that is, if Input I becomes positive with respect to Input II, there is a downward deflection.)

In the simplest example, consider a spike with a very limited potential field involving only T4 (Figure 1-9). The electrode pairs in this case are F8 → T4, and T4 → T6. The display or write out of the electrical activity from each electrode pair is known as a Channel. F8 → T4 could be termed Channel 1, and T4 → T6 Channel 2. In this case, the adjacent channels containing the T4 electrode record the same potential but in opposite directions. This creates the phase reversal. Recall that most spike discharges at the surface are negative in sign.

Note that in Channel 1 T4 is in Input II. Input II suddenly becomes negative with respect to Input I by 80 μV, resulting in a downward deflection (the opposite of the rule). In Channel 2, T4 is in Input I. The same spike causes Input I to become negative with respect to Input II by the same 80 μV. Thus, the spike will be recorded as an upward deflection. Remember, Channels 1 and 2 are displaying the same potential but with opposite deflections. Again, this is the phase reversal – the localization principle of bipolar recording.

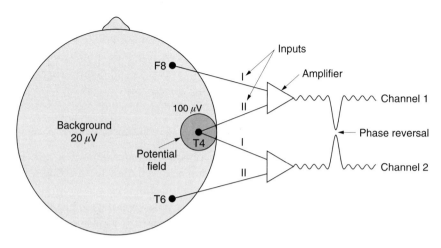

**Figure 1-9** Principle of bipolar localization. The figure depicts a spike discharge of 100 μV at T4. The potential is conducted to Input II in the first amplifier, and to Input I in the second amplifier. Other electrodes are not affected by the event. The result is known as a phase reversal.

Let us now analyze the display when a spike at F8 has a wider potential field that also affects T4 (Figure 1-10).

In Channel 1, the voltage at F8 (100 μV) is compared with the lower voltage at Fp2 (50 μV). Because F8 is in Input II, a downward deflection of 50 μV (100 μV – 50 μV) will be recorded.

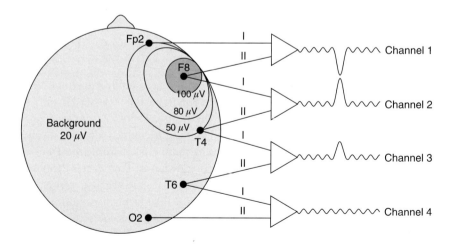

**Figure 1-10** Here, a spike discharge of 100 μV at F8 spreads to involve Fp2 and T4, each at 50 μV. The potential difference between F8 and the other two electrodes is 50 μV. The display demonstrates a phase reversal at F8 (Channels 1 and 2) with representation of the spike in Channel 3 (the potential difference between T4 and T6 is 30 μV).

In Channel 2, the voltage at F8 is compared to the lower voltage at T4. Because F8 in this case is in Input I, an upward deflection of 50 μV will be recorded (the same potential difference as in Channel 1).

In Channel 3, the lower potential recorded at T4 (50 μV) is compared to T6, which is unaffected by the F8 spike but is recording the background activity (at an average of 20 μV). Because T4 is in Input I, an upward deflection of 30 μV (50 μV − 20 μV) will be recorded.

In Channel 4, the voltage at T6 is compared with O2. Both are unaffected by the F8 spike. There is no potential difference, and thus no deflection.

Other channels, for example F4 → C4 and C4 → P4 may be affected by the declining potential field generated at F8. Thus, phase reversals at lower amplitude would be recorded at these sites. Note that these considerations apply to any potential at any point on the scalp.

## Referential Recording

In referential recording the amplifiers are not linked as in bipolar recording. Signals from each of the scalp electrodes (known as exploring electrodes) are conducted to Input I of the associated amplifier, while signals from the reference are conducted to Input II. Thus, in referential recording, we record the potential difference between a particular scalp electrode and a referential electrode. Theoretically, the reference can be located anywhere, but there are practical considerations. A reference placed at any distant point will be contaminated with 60 Hz artifact (50 Hz in Europe). A reference placed on, say, the shoulder or chest would also pick up high-voltage EKG artifact. Interference from both these factors would render the EEG unreadable. The ears are relatively free from both these artifacts, although it must be said that EKG is sometimes a contaminant at the ear electrodes. Moreover, due to the proximity of the ears to T3/T4 electrodes, the ears do pick up cerebral activity from these locations.

Now, utilizing the ears as ipsilateral references, let us compare the voltage of an event occurring at F4 with that at an ipsilateral ear reference, A2 (Figure 1-11). In this example we will assume that A2 is neutral at 0 μV. Here we have a spike discharge with an amplitude of 100 μV. The potential field of the spike spreads to C4 with an amplitude of 70 μV, and to P4 with an amplitude of 30 μV. Beyond these points there is no representation of the field associated with the spike.

In referential recording, the localization principle is amplitude. That is, the exploring electrode recording the greatest amplitude of the wave in question, in this case a spike at F4, defines the focus (Figure 1-11).

We now present the paradox of bipolar recording. The paradox is a result of the above mentioned in-phase cancellation – that is, potentials that are equal in the two inputs of an amplifier are not represented in the display. In other words, there is no potential difference! The unwary, when examining Channels 2 and 3 of Figure 1-12A, might conclude that little if anything is occurring at F8, T4,

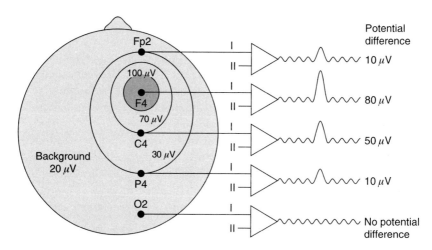

**Figure 1-11** Principle of referential localization. A spike discharge of 100 μV at F4 spreads to involve Fp2, C4 and P4. The potential at the active electrodes is conducted to Input I of each amplifier. Output from the reference is conducted to Input II. Note that the amplitude of the displayed spike is proportional to the voltage at each active electrode.

and T6. On the other hand, when one looks at the same situation with referential recording, it becomes clear that the maximum abnormality underlies those very electrodes (Figure 1-12B).

References other than the ears are also in common use. One is the vertex (Cz), often used in a referential montage to complement the ear reference. The astute reader will recognize that the vertex resides in a sea of cerebral activity. Thus, the background of the EEG recorded by the vertex electrode will be referred to Input II of all channels. As long as this is recognized, one is able to determine the location of a waveform that stands out from the background (e.g. a spike or delta wave).

A note on ear and vertex referential recording: A recorded event (spike, slow wave) is best represented when the reference is distant from the exploring electrode. Considering the ipsilateral ear reference (A1 or A2), the ear is close to the midtemporal electrode (T3 or T4). On the other hand, the paracentral electrodes are farther away from the reference. Thus, a spike at T3 or T4, the field of which also affects A1 and A2, will be recorded at lower amplitude than a spike at an electrode more distant from the reference. Conversely, when recording with a vertex reference, the potential field of a spike recorded at one of the temporal electrodes, far from Cz, is unlikely to affect this reference and thus will be well represented. By the same token, a spike at C3 or C4 would be less well defined when using a Cz reference. These features do not create a problem if the principle of localization is recalled (amplitude), and if both vertex and ear references are utilized during the recording. In other words, the ear and vertex references are complimentary.

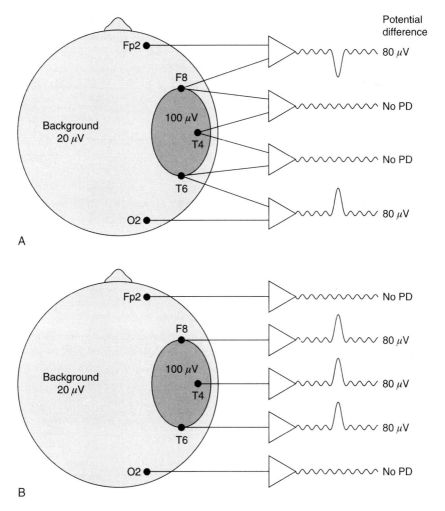

**Figure 1-12** The paradox of bipolar recording. (A) Representation of a 100 μV spike that affects F8, T4, and T6 equally. Inasmuch as there is no potential difference between F8→T4 and T4 → T6, the spike is not recorded in Channels 2 and 3 and gives the impression that there is no abnormality at T4. (B) Same discharge in referential recording. Note equal deflections in Channels 2, 3, and 4. The true picture is thus displayed.

A widely used reference is the common average reference. In this scheme, the voltage of an event occurring under a particular electrode (the exploring electrode) is compared to the average voltage recorded by all the electrodes on the scalp, conducted through high resistance. This creates a situation in which a focal spike discharge, say confined to F7, will result in an upward deflection at F7 (Input I), and downward deflections in many of the other channels (remember – the reference, in this case the average of activity from all the electrodes, is in

Input II – see the RULE, page 11). Because activity from all channels is averaged, the effect of any one channel on the remainder is relatively small. If, on the other hand, the potential field involves other electrodes (as it usually does), there will be upward deflections at those points with amplitudes proportional to the recorded voltage, and downward deflections at the other non-involved electrodes. Note that the upward deflections thus recorded define the potential field of the event (Figure 1-13).

## Montage Selection

Montage refers to the pattern of systematic linkage of the scalp electrodes designed to obtain a logical display of the electrical activity. Unlike the 10-20 system of electrode placement described above, there is no international standard of montages to be used in EEG laboratories. Certain montages, however, are in widespread use. In bipolar recording the anterior-posterior (A-P) arrangement is perhaps the most popular (known in the trade as the "double banana," and by some as the Queen Square montage) (Figure 1-14).

**Note**: arrows are often used in North America for convenience: the tail of the arrow indicates Input I; the point of the arrow Input II.

Adjacent electrodes are connected from front to back, including the temporal chain (some call this the low line) and the paracentral or supra-Sylvian chain (some say high line). The EEG is displayed in various ways. In this example, the

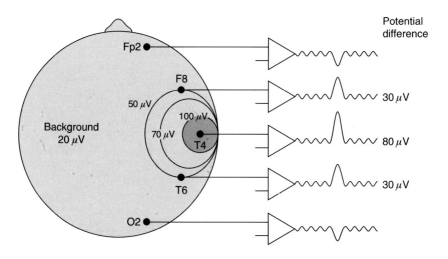

**Figure 1-13** Common average recording of a spike discharge of 100 μV at T4, spreading to involve F8 and T6. In Channels 2, 3, and 4 the amplitude is proportional to the recorded voltage (potential difference between the active electrodes (in Input I) and the average reference (in Input II). Note the downward deflections at lower voltage in Channels 1 and 5, reflecting the attenuated voltage represented by the average of all the electrodes on the scalp.

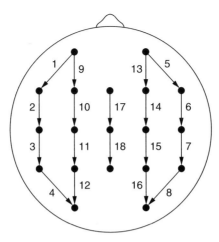

**Figure 1-14** A typical anterior-posterior montage of bipolar recording. The numbers refer to channels, odd on the left and even on the right. Both temporal and supra-Sylvian chains alternate from left to right. The arrows represent the inputs to each amplifier. The tail is in Input I and the point in Input II.

four channels of the low line on one side are followed by the four low line channels on the opposite side. Similarly, the four channels of the high line also alternate. In North America, the left side is written out first followed by the right. In Europe the opposite is the case. Some laboratories write out the eight channels of left-sided electrodes followed by the right-sided electrodes. Still others prefer alternating homologous channels, for example Fp1 → F7; Fp2 → F8, and so on. Overall, the latter tends to be a bit more confusing – but electroencephalographers experienced with a particular electrode arrangement have no difficulty.

A second popular arrangement is the transverse montage. This links adjacent electrodes in transverse chains, starting anteriorly and progressing posteriorly. Each chain starts with the left side and progresses to the right (e.g. F7 → F3 → Fz → F4 → F8). The transverse montage is particularly well suited to record abnormalities occurring at or near the vertex (e.g. midline spikes) (Figure 1-15).

With respect to referential recording, the recording is usually displayed in both A-P and transverse arrangements, reprising commonly used bipolar montages. A variety of other montages are employed at the discretion of the individual electroencephalographer. The idea, in short, is to highlight certain areas of interest in the best possible way. Two additional montages come to mind: the circle or hatband, and the inferior coronal. The circle montage connects electrodes through the fronto-polar and occipital electrodes, traveling over the temporal regions. Frontal and occipital activities are thus well displayed. The inferior coronal montage, traversing central and mid-temporal locations to the ears, connecting the ears, is useful in bringing out low-voltage temporal abnormalities. If the student is familiar with the 10-20 system and is apprised of the montage, he or she should have no difficulty in interpreting the record.

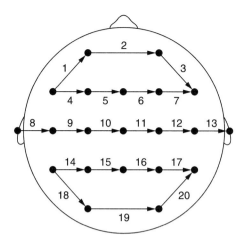

**Figure 1-15** A possible transverse montage of bipolar recording. The chains run from left to right, beginning anteriorly and proceeding posteriorly. Note that the midline electrodes are incorporated into the second, third, and fourth chains, thus allowing good representation of midline events.

In the era of digital EEG, specific montage selection by the technologist is not as critical as it was in the past. All recording is actually done referentially. The software allows display of recorded potentials in any desired montage. Thus, the technician and reader can now easily switch from one montage to another to examine the characteristics of a particular phenomenon. A low-amplitude temporal spike during bipolar recording can rapidly be inspected on a referential montage with the flick of the computer mouse. Regardless of technological developments, however, the underlying principles remain the same.

In summary, the electroencephalographer selects the sequence of montages to be used by the technologist but this should allow him or her to alter the sequence or the duration of recording in a particular montage to suit the clinical problem. Remember, the central idea is to maximize the opportunity to display an abnormality for optimal recognition.

**Overview of Electronics**

We often say that the EEG display can be manipulated at will and made to demonstrate a severe abnormality, or to show a normal pattern. This manipulation refers to changing the electronic circuitry with the press of a button (or use of a mouse) in order to alter sensitivity, filtration, and write-out or display speed. Clearly, some order was required so that EEGs obtained in one laboratory are easily interpretable at another. For many years nearly all laboratories in North America, and indeed in many laboratories throughout the world, have used similar electronic settings for routine work. Following is a brief discussion of the most important recording parameters.

### Calibration

A square-wave signal injected into the recording system that indicates the response of the write-out system to a given voltage. With paper systems, a signal of 50 μV is injected to all channels by a control on the EEG machine producing a deflection of 7 mm. The recorded waveform rapidly decays in amplitude due to the system's high pass filter (see below). All paper EEG recordings should include at the beginning a calibration signal for each channel. At the end of recording, calibration should also be recorded, including those associated with different sensitivities used during recording. With digital systems, standard calibration is automatic. There is no need for multiple calibration signals at the end of recording due to the fact that the reader selects differential sensitivities at will while reading the record.

### Display (write-out)

In most North American and many European laboratories the standard display speed is 30 mm/sec with 10 seconds of EEG per display or page. There is nothing magic about the number – in fact, some laboratories (particularly in Europe) prefer a speed of 15 mm/sec. The appearance of the EEG is considerably altered in the latter case (e.g. the alpha rhythm looks like rhythmic beta activity). The important point is that the reader knows what speed is selected. It should be said that there are instances when use of a slower speed is quite useful, for example in the identification of periodicity, or even rhythmicity of a particular phenomenon. Likewise, increasing write out speed to, say, 60 mm/sec may allow one to analyze more accurately wave configuration, particularly when a phenomenon is "crowded" as in grouped spikes. With digital EEG the display speed is easily changed with the mouse to suit the reader's needs.

### Sensitivity

The sensitivity of each channel refers to the amplitude of the display produced by the received signal. The measurement is expressed in voltage per deflection. Standard sensitivity is 7 μV/mm.

Sensitivity may be altered for any particular channel depending on the specific need. For example, the sensitivity of a channel recording the EKG or EOG would have to be decreased due to the much higher voltage of these signals (measured in millivolts). In general, the sensitivity of all channels recording the EEG may be changed simultaneously by a stepped gain control. For example, one might wish to increase sensitivity in situations where the general voltage of the EEG is low. Similarly, some EEG phenomena reach very high voltages, for example generalized spike-wave discharges, requiring a decrease in sensitivity in order properly to analyze the waveforms.

### Low-pass (high-frequency, HF) filters

This is a resistance/capacitance circuit that progressively attenuates undesirable high frequencies, for example muscle action potentials. In addition, a notch filter setting of 60 Hz is usually employed, reducing 60 Hz interference. The standard HF setting is 70 Hz: high-frequency signals (e.g. beta activity or rapid spikes) are only mildly attenuated. Note that attenuation varies as the recorded frequency differs from the filter setting. Other standard settings are 35 Hz and 15 Hz, the latter severely attenuating a broad range of high frequencies. As a practical matter, recording at a HF setting of 15 Hz should not be employed save in rare and unusual circumstances. An unwanted consequence would be a marked attenuation of spike potentials.

Unfortunately, the authors have inspected EEGs from outside sources in which a HF setting of 15 Hz was used throughout. Such records look "clean," but fail to convey needed information. Don't do it.

### High-pass (low-frequency) filters

This is also known as the time constant (TC) and is a resistance/capacitance circuit that attenuates low frequencies. The decline in response is exponential and is termed the TC, that is, the time in seconds required for the signal to attenuate by 37 percent of its original value. Standard recording is carried out at a TC of 0.3 second or 1.0 second. At higher TCs there is marked attenuation of slow potentials, with little effect on rapid potentials such as spikes.

### Notes on Recording the EEG

Many special problems confront the technologist in his or her efforts to obtain an EEG that successfully can be interpreted by the electroencephalographer. We emphasize that the electroencephalographer is totally dependent on the quality of the recording – that is, regardless of the expertise of the reader, he or she is unable to use that expertise in the face of a technically inadequate tracing. For example, elimination or reduction of artifact is largely the responsibility of the technologist. The ability properly to place electrodes in conformity with the 10-20 International System (including, importantly, accurate measurements of electrode location) is critical if one is to compare electrical activity between the two hemispheres with accuracy. The technologist must also be conversant with the basic elements of the patient's history and be able to tailor-make the record to the patient's particular problem. As an example, if epilepsy is suspected, the technologist should attempt to record drowsiness, and sleep if possible. Only so much can be done, but ensuring a calm, quiet and supportive environment goes a long way. Moreover, since focal epileptiform activity is often activated by the interface between wake and drowsiness, the technologist should gently alert the drowsy patient on several occasions in an attempt to provoke latent spikes. A clue may be provided by the waking record – perhaps a few episodic or paroxysmal temporal theta waves during wakefulness will blossom into sharp waves or spikes during drowsiness. At the other end of the spectrum, if a patient is sleeping at the onset of the test, he or she should be aroused after some minutes of recording. This ensures that a relative waking record is obtained. Unfortunately, sleep may obscure background abnormalities that are only evident when the patient is awake – a circumstance sometimes encountered in patients with dementia.

With respect to the above comments, and after the student has participated in actual recordings, it will become clear that the most important player in providing the clinician with reliable diagnostic information is the technologist. He or she begins to become proficient after about six months in the laboratory, and the best gain in expertise over the course of years. Indeed, a successful, diagnostically useful recording is a collaborative effort between technologist and interpreter.

## ARTIFACTS

Recognition of artifacts is one of the vexing aspects of EEG interpretation and also one of the most important. As a beginner, you may find the differentiation of artifacts from physiological phenomena quite difficult. We note that the archeologist loves artifacts and spends a lifetime searching for them. On the other hand, the electroencephalographer hates them, tends to criticize the technicians when artifacts mar the record, and gives young readers a bad time when they do not recognize them. A distinguishing characteristic of the experienced electroencephalographer is the ability reliably to recognize artifacts. For the most part the reader will soon master artifact recognition, particularly after understanding their characteristics and referring to the mini-atlas, and should not be too daunted by the seeming impossibility of this task!

Artifacts come in many different forms and have diverse causes. The major underlying problem is the enormous amplification required to record brain waves. As a result, amplified non-cerebral potentials – for example vigorous movements by the patient producing random excursions of the electrode leads – may render the EEG uninterpretable. Other specific artifacts requiring recognition are detailed below:

Electrode "pop": An important source of artifacts is faulty electrode contact resulting in the electrode "pop" (A-24). In such cases slight movement of the head disturbs an already poor contact of the scalp electrode, resulting in a sudden momentary increase in electrode impedance. The extracerebral potential is referred to the offending electrode. In bipolar recording the resultant phase reversal is an exact mirror image referable to the common electrode in adjacent channels. In referential recording, only one channel reflects the "pop." In both cases there is no potential field. Continual electrode artifact is also encountered, rendering that portion of the record unsatisfactory (A-25).

**Muscle action potentials**: Nearly all EEGs contain muscle artifact. When excessive, it impairs our ability to interpret the EEG adequately. Muscle artifact is commonly maximal in the frontal and temporal regions due to electrode placement over the frontalis and temporalis muscles. If the technician asks the patient to open his or her mouth slightly, thus relaxing the jaw, muscle artifact from the temporal regions may be reduced. At times, isolated muscle action potentials may be mistaken for spike discharges. An important differential point is the duration of the muscle potential, which is less than 20 ms (spike potentials have durations of 20–80 ms). It is sometimes possible to discern abnormal cerebral potentials beneath muscle artifact. For example, underlying slow waves (particularly delta waves) may be evident. Thus, the presence of muscle artifact does not necessarily preempt rendering a verdict of abnormality.

**Chewing artifact**: Generalized muscle action potentials that have a rhythmicity coincident with repetitive chewing motions (A-28).

**Tongue movement artifact**: Slow, random potentials resembling delta waves. The inconsistency of the potential fields gives a clue to the artifactual nature of the apparent slowing (A-30).

**Perspiration artifact**: Very slow, undulating potentials having durations of several seconds (A-31). The artifact reflects "shorting" of currents between electrodes owing to a marked reduction of electrode impedance. In this case the salt-rich perspiration creates what is known as a salt bridge.

**Various rhythmic frequencies** (e.g. alpha or theta range, confined to a single electrode): May be difficult to differentiate from ictal activity. The artifact is secondary to poor electrode contact. There is no potential field, and the frequency is recorded only in two adjacent channels in bipolar and one channel in referential recording.

**ECG artifact**: Sharp potentials coincident with the ECG (A-23). EEGs usually reserve one channel for ECG, thus ensuring easy recognition of this artifact. The artifact is particularly prominent in channels connected to the ears. It also may be diffuse. If there is no ECG monitor, and if the patient has atrial fibrillation or frequent premature contractions, the artifact may be confounding, inconsistent, and masquerade as spike discharges. Look for phase relationships that do not comport with those of true spikes. ECG artifact is particularly prominent in the obese and those with hypertension.

**Movement artifact**: Random, wide excursions of recorders coincident with body or head movements and associated with muscle artifact. Such movements alter the positions of the leads and may also change the contact between the electrodes and the skin.

**IV artifact**: Periodic potentials in one or more channels coincident with the intravenous (IV) drip (A-29). May be confusing if the technician fails to inform the electroencephalographer of the presence of an IV near the leads. The charge on the droplet is thought responsible.

**Feeding pump artifact**: A mechanical artifact resulting from a feeding pump. The artifact is rhythmic and may be quite sharp, giving the impression of an ictal focus. Accurate notations by the technician are key in sorting out this unusual phenomenon (A-36).

**Respirator artifact**: Wide, usually high-amplitude excursions that may resemble delta waves (A-32). A check on the rhythmicity (usually in the range of 12 per min), along with a stereotyped waveform, makes the diagnosis. Note that the artifact may be of relatively low voltage and, in cases where the patient overrides the respirator, demonstrate irregularity. In this circumstance, differentiation from intermittent electrocortical delta activity may be a problem. The technologist can save the day by marking the respirations on the record.

**LVAD and IBP artifacts**: LVAD (left ventricular assist device); IBP (Intra-aortic balloon counterpulsation). These devices, used to assist patients with severe congestive heart failure or for patients awaiting heart transplant, produce a high-voltage sharp, rhythmic artifact in all leads. In most cases the record is rendered uninterpretable (A-33).

**Pulse artifact**: A rhythmic, sharply contoured waveform at the same frequency as ECG. The rise time is faster than the fall time. This artifact arises when an electrode is placed over a scalp artery, for example a branch of the superficial temporal artery. Displacing the electrode just away from the artery (say, 1–2 cm) should eliminate the artifact.

**60 Hz artifact**: Rhythmic frequency at 60 Hz (or 50 Hz) secondary to nearby electrical apparatus or poor grounding, usually expressed because of high electrode impedance but sometimes difficult to eliminate. Particularly problematic in ICU settings where many electrical devices are in use. It sometimes is possible to alter the position of visible wiring, or even to turn off a monitor temporarily (with permission, of course) in an attempt to reduce the artifact. Proper grounding is always helpful.

**Eye blink artifact**: High-voltage potentials, maximal in the frontal derivations (A-26). The deviations are synchronous with a major downward deflection. The display results from the corneoretinal potential (the cornea is electropositive with respect to the retina, measured in millivolts), along with a minor contribution of the electroretinogram (ERG). During an eyeblink the globes turn slightly upward (Bell's phenomenon). Thus, the fronto-polar electrodes become momentarily positive. (Recall the rule concerning deflections; see page 11.) Eyelid-flutter produces a rhythmic bifrontal frequency at 8 to 10 Hz.

Sometimes a patient has a prosthetic eye; in this situation, the artifact is expressed on only one side (A-35). One will also see limited eye blink potentials in those with a third nerve palsy.

**Lateral eye movement artifact**: Recognizable in the fronto-temporal derivations as sharply contoured potentials that are out of phase (A-27). For example, if the eyes deviate to the left, the globe on the left approaches the left anterior temporal electrode (F7) while the right globe turns away from the right anterior temporal electrode (F8). A positive potential is therefore recorded at F7 and a negative potential at F8. (Remember, the cornea is positive with respect to the retina.) Thus, in bipolar recording, the resultant waveforms deviate away from each other in the two channels connected to F7, while the opposite is the case with the channels connected to F8. If the patient has nystagmus, the potentials are rhythmic and rapid, coincident with nystagmus frequency. Note also that very rapid spike potentials may occur during lateral eye movements with potential maxima at the F7/F8 electrodes. These result from movements of the lateral rectus muscles and are known as lateral rectus spikes.

**Roving eye movements**: Slow, lateral eye movements during drowsiness that produce slow waves with alternating phase relationships in the fronto-temporal derivations (A-34).

**Tremor artifact**: A usually rhythmic frequency, often most evident in the posterior derivations. Repetitive movements of a limb are transmitted to the head, resulting in subtle oscillations affecting the occipital electrodes. A typical example is the 5 to 6 Hz tremor of Parkinsonism. For the unwary, the artifact can resemble a rhythmic seizure discharge. The technician should indicate the presence of clinical tremor and add an electromyogram (EMG) electrode for clarity.

**Walking artifact**: Personnel walking near the patient during an ICU or bedside recording can produce a rhythmic artifact resembling a sharp wave discharge (A-37).

**Shiver artifact**: Bursts of rhythmic widespread sharp potentials, contaminated with muscle artifact, at a frequency of 10 to 14 Hz. Again, documentation by the technician is important for recognition.

**Patting artifact**: Rhythmic potentials resembling an ictal discharge, usually produced by a mother who holds her baby on her lap during the EEG (A-38).

**Suck artifact**: Seen in infants. May be rapid and highly rhythmic with various waveforms. Could be mistaken for an ictal discharge. The technician should note when the infant is sucking.

**Sob artifact**: Seen in infants. Irregular and repetitive slow potentials. Again, the technician should note when sobs occur.

# 2

---

# THE NORMAL EEG

## THE NORMAL ADULT EEG

Understanding the elements of the normal EEG is a prerequisite for developing expertise in interpreting the abnormal record. In the following discussion, the frequency bands and individual waveforms found in the normal adult EEG are described for both the waking (A-1) and sleeping states.

### The Alpha Rhythm

Hans Berger, the Berlin psychiatrist who in 1929 first described the EEG in man, named the first rhythmic frequency he discovered the alpha. The alpha in fact is the principal background feature of the normal adult EEG. It is defined as a rhythmic frequency at 8 to 13 Hz, usually of maximal amplitude in the occipital regions. Alpha is best seen when the person is in the relaxed, waking state with eyes closed. Another feature is its attenuation with eye opening, and return when the eyes are closed. Note that waves in the alpha frequency band may be found in various locations and in various states (e.g. alpha coma or evolution of an epileptic discharge). Such waves are not the alpha as described above.

The alpha is sometimes referred to as the posterior dominant rhythm (PDR). The PDR, however, may be in slower frequency bands, for example in children or in the presence of diffuse disease processes. This will be discussed in subsequent sections.

We will now describe the alpha in considerable detail with respect to its amplitude, symmetry, abundance, distribution, variability, and changes with alterations in state of awareness. This is important not only for the alpha itself but also gives a clue to how other frequencies may be evaluated. If you are confident about describing the alpha, you will be more confident about the EEG in general. Thus, for example, you will be in a good position to evaluate activities associated with sleep, their distribution, how they change with stimulation, and changes associated with age.

In assessing alpha, look for the patient's best – that is, the highest posterior frequency achieved during the most alert state. Slower posterior rhythms in the theta range or theta waves admixed with the alpha may be due to mild drowsiness and thus have no pathological significance.

Alpha is usually more or less symmetrical but often is of higher amplitude over the non-dominant hemisphere. In that case a 2:1 ratio is acceptable; if greater than 2:1, it becomes a matter for consideration. It may be related to an abnormality, but it also could be the result of incorrect electrode placement. The latter is more likely if the lower-amplitude alpha is well organized and equally persistent as that on the opposite side. Consideration might be given to the possible presence of an insulating process between the scalp electrodes and the cerebral cortex, as might be seen with a subdural collection. In that case the alpha on the affected side may either be markedly depressed in amplitude, or absent.

Alpha, while usually maximal in the occipital regions, often distributes to the adjacent parietal and posterior temporal areas. Moreover, this may be variable over the course of the recording. The spread of alpha may not be symmetrical. Thus, when determining alpha symmetry, or lack thereof, the reader should visually average parietal/occipital and posterior temporal/occipital alpha over the two hemispheres. In some cases, alpha may spread more widely without obvious significance. Rarely, frontal alpha is encountered in a neurologically unimpaired person.

If alpha increases in frequency when the patient opens his or her eyes and persists with the eyes open, or appears only during eye-opening, drowsiness is a likely cause. These features are sometimes noted in patients with dementia. Some normal persons have little or no alpha during the resting state. This finding has no clinical significance and occurs in perhaps 5 percent of individuals. If the patient is tense, alpha may not be recorded. In such cases, alpha may appear during hyperventilation as the patient becomes more relaxed.

Take note of processes that may lead to a decline in alpha frequency. These include (but are not limited to) effect of medication(s) such as phenytoin or psychotropic drugs, early dementias, increased intracranial pressure, hypothyroidism, and other metabolic disorders such as hepatic insufficiency (see sections dealing with these conditions).

The absence of alpha on one side is always pathological. In older subjects this asymmetry is often due to remote infarction. In younger subjects the cause is more likely to be brain damage such as congenital hemiatrophy. If a record contains apparent alpha and looks relatively normal, save for the fact that the alpha frequency is prominent in the frontal regions, interpretation depends on the state of the patient. In a comatose patient (e.g. after cardiopulmonary arrest), it is termed alpha coma and carries a dismal prognosis (see section on Coma).

## Beta Activity

Beta activity is defined as a frequency of 14 Hz and above. Beta, the second waveform described by Berger, is rhythmic in character and is present in the background of most subjects. If completely absent it may represent an abnormality depending on other features of the EEG (see below). Beta must be differentiated from muscle action potentials. The latter may be rhythmic or arrhythmic but have briefer durations than beta waves. Beta varies greatly in amplitude, even in the absence of factors such as medication. This feature generally is of little consequence.

Maximal beta amplitude is usually in the frontocentral regions, but it may be widespread. It does not respond to eye opening, as does the alpha. During drowsiness, beta may seem to increase in amplitude. This appears to be a function of amplitude diminution of other background frequencies and thus is more apparent than real.

Beta activity increases in amplitude and abundance by various drugs, for example barbiturates, chloral hydrate, benzodiazepines, and tricyclic antidepressants (A-22) (see section on Medication Effects). In fact, excessive beta in the EEG tends to impair accurate interpretation of the record. Attempts have been made to correlate beta frequency with various classes of drugs, but little useful clinical information has resulted.

Perhaps the most important finding when analyzing beta activity is interhemispheric asymmetry. In particular, the side of reduced amplitude usually points to the pathological hemisphere. Examples include remote infarct, subdural collections, and porencephaly. By the same token, beta amplitude may be unilaterally increased. This occurs in a setting of a previous craniotomy (so-called breach rhythm) (A-57). Increased amplitude may also occur over the site of a brain tumor. Beta asymmetry, if present, should always be considered in concert with asymmetry of other background frequencies.

## Theta Activity

Theta activity (4–7 Hz) is usually present in the waking adult EEG, although it may be completely absent. It tends to be somewhat more evident in the midline and temporal derivations. Some authors think the normal adult waking EEG should contain no more than about 5 percent theta, though this is quite variable. In any event, be certain that the subject is actually awake, or the theta may simply reflect early drowsiness. It should be symmetrically distributed.

If theta activity is found in only one location, or is predominant over one hemisphere, it is likely to reflect underlying structural disease. The lesion, however, is usually less malignant, or extensive, than in the case of delta-range focality. Examples are meningioma, low-grade glioma, and remote infarction. Focal theta is sometimes non-pathological, especially when it appears as a rhythmic frequency in one or both mid-temporal regions. In this case the theta is considered a normal variant (see section on this topic).

Diffuse theta is usual in children. In the young, theta abundance is quite variable, and one should be flexible when determining whether the theta is excessive or not. When in doubt, err on the side of normality. In comatose patients who have suffered catastrophic brain damage, rhythmic theta may be found in the frontal regions. This finding is termed theta coma and has the same significance as alpha coma (see section on Coma).

## Delta Activity

Delta activity (< 4 Hz) was described in 1936 by W. Gray Walter, a young English physiologist. He gathered his bulky EEG apparatus in an operating room where a patient was undergoing neurosurgery for a malignant tumor. Electrodes placed over the involved area recorded very slow, high-voltage potentials that were slower in frequency than previously reported waveforms. Walter termed these potentials delta waves. Since that time, focal delta activity has proved a reliable indicator of localized disease of the brain.

As a rule, delta waves are not present in the normal adult waking, resting record. It follows that their presence implies cerebral dysfunction. We emphasize the waking record inasmuch as delta is an important component of sleep in adults. It also may occur in elderly subjects in relatively limited amounts, particularly in the temporal regions. Such slowing, while probably indicating some degree of cerebral pathology, for example vascular disease, does not necessarily imply focal lesions that are demonstrable in imaging studies.

There are other circumstances wherein delta is a normal component of the EEG. For instance, delta is prominent in infants and young children (see section on EEG in children), and is common in adolescents in the posterior head regions (posterior slow waves of youth, A-7).

Delta may occur diffusely (implying a diffuse cerebral process), or it may be recorded as rhythmic waves in the frontal or other head regions. The latter have a particular significance (see section on projected rhythms). Finally, delta may be of very high voltage, implying severe or acute dysfunction, or of very low voltage, as in a patient with depressed consciousness. These issues will be discussed in subsequent sections.

## Mu Rhythm

Mu rhythm, sometimes called wicket rhythm, is a normal finding (A-10). It is found in the central derivations (C3/C4) over the motor strip. It may be unilateral or bilateral; if bilateral it may be synchronous or asynchronous. Its name derives from the waveform – a sharply contoured, rhythmic frequency at 7 to 11 Hz resembling the Greek letter. Mu is sometimes more evident during drowsiness, and during recording with eyes open. It is considered to be related to beta activity, possibly a subharmonic. Mu attenuates with movement of the opposite upper limb (e.g. making a fist), or even thinking about such an action. It often is prominent over the site of a craniotomy. The importance of mu lies mainly in its recognition as a normal finding. **Note**: mu rhythm is to be differentiated from wicket spikes (see section on normal variants).

## Lambda Waves

Lambda waves are electropositive transients recorded in the occipital regions (A-11). They are sharply contoured, usually symmetrical, and can be mistaken for epileptiform potentials. At the same time, lambda often goes unnoticed due to lack of awareness by the reader as well as the absence of circumstances, which lead to their expression, namely scanning eye movements. Having the subject look at a picture containing interesting subjects or details may provoke lambda waves. One of the authors has used a photograph depicting the Knights of the Round Table, first used by Bickford (for many years a foremost electroencephalographer at the Mayo Clinic), to generate lambda waves. The subject automatically scans this interesting setting, and lambda waves become prominent. Lambda waves probably represent visual evoked potentials. Again, the principal advantage to recognizing lambda is the knowledge that it is a normal finding and not an example of epileptiform activity.

### Features of Sleep

The recording of sleep is one of the most powerful diagnostic adjuncts in electroencephalography. Relatively minor abnormalities on the routine EEG may be amplified during sleep, and new abnormalities may appear. This is particularly the case with epileptiform activity. Most patients become drowsy at some point during a routine recording, and many actually sleep spontaneously for variable periods. Focal spike or sharp wave discharges often appear or are increased during Stage I sleep (drowsiness) and Stage II sleep.

Likewise, focal slow wave abnormalities may be exaggerated during these stages. With deeper sleep (slow wave sleep, SWS) there is a tendency for epileptiform activity and focal slowing to become less obvious.

Stage I sleep is characterized by slowing, fragmentation (increasing irregularity), and ultimate disappearance of the alpha or the posterior dominant rhythm (PDR, A-12). In some cases the PDR disappears abruptly. The background may appear to be generally of lower voltage (due to absence of the PDR), and beta activity may be more obvious. Diffuse theta activity appears and increases in abundance. In older patients delta waves may be admixed with the theta frequencies. Bifrontal delta waves are common in older subjects. Stage I may also contain early elements of Stage II, for example vertex sharp waves, K-complexes, Positive Occipital Sharp Transients of Sleep (POSTS) and even brief, poorly developed sleep spindles (see definitions below). Note that surprisingly rapid cycling between wakefulness (W) and Stage I sleep is not unusual.

Stage II sleep arrives with the appearance of well-defined sleep spindles – synchronous, rhythmic waves at 12 to 14 ($\pm$ 2) Hz with a potential maximum in the central regions (A-14). Amplitude varies and is of little importance. If only fragmentary or very brief, transient spindles are recorded, the patient is not considered to be firmly in Stage II. In addition, there is increased diffuse slowing both in theta and delta ranges. Other elements of sleep become more prominent, in particular vertex sharp waves (V-waves) and K-complexes. Vertex sharp waves are synchronous, episodic, sharply contoured potentials that are maximal over the central regions (A-13). They may assume a very sharp, spike-like configuration, are variable in amplitude, and sometimes occur in rhythmic runs. K-complexes are high-voltage, synchronous bi- or triphasic slow potentials with a bifrontal or central preponderance, often (but not invariably) in close association with sleep spindles. In addition, POSTS may be quite prominent (A-15). These potentials have the appearance of sharp waves, are electropositive at the occipital electrodes, and may be mono- or biphasic in configuration. Do not be surprised to find long rhythmic runs of POSTS that could be mistaken for an ictal discharge by the unwary.

SWS is characterized by increasing amounts of diffuse delta activity, and is clearly established when more than 50 percent of the record is taken up with delta. At the same time there is a progressive decline in sleep spindles – in fact, they may disappear. The delta may reach very high voltage without clinical significance. In adults, SWS is seldom encountered during routine recording.

Rapid eye movement (REM) sleep is seen infrequently in adults. Recall that the first REM period usually occurs about 90 minutes after sleep onset. An exception is the patient with narcolepsy who experiences REM onset sleep. When REM sleep is recorded, the eye channels (recording from electrodes placed just above and lateral to the eyes), as well as the Fp1-F7 and Fp2-F8 derivations, demonstrate irregular vertical and horizontal eye movements. The EEG background consists of low-voltage theta activity.

## SPECIAL CONSIDERATIONS IN CHILDREN

In order to understand the EEG in children we emphasize that variability is the rule – certainly much greater than in adults. This applies to the background rhythmic activity as well as to the presence of generalized irregular slow waves. There is a steady increase in the frequency of the posterior dominant rhythm as the child matures. The rate of increase is highly variable, reflecting, it is presumed, differential rates of brain maturation.

Posterior rhythmic activity is not present at birth, but begins to appear in the second or third month of life. Initially rhythmic delta waves predominate, but soon a polyrhythmic pattern develops consisting of delta and theta components. There is a gradual increase in average frequency (A-2), with slow theta range activity predominating by one year. Note that many admixed delta components will be present. By age 3 years, one sees fairly well-established rhythmic theta. Sometimes a small amount of alpha activity is intermingled and delta is much less evident (A-3, A-4). By age 6 years alpha is usually quite well established. The alpha frequency increases thereafter, reaching an average of 10 Hz by age 7 to 8 years or so (A-5). We emphasize that this progression represents a general statement that applies to many normals. Some delay in reaching the alpha range is not in and of itself abnormal. When in doubt, opt for a declaration of normal rather than abnormal.

The next task is assessment of generalized slowing. Our students often ask: how much slowing is too much? When can one say that the amount of slowing indicates some degree of bilateral cerebral dysfunction? We believe that it is prudent to be fairly generous when making this determination. During the first year of life there is a gradual shift of generalized slowing from delta to theta. Over the next two years, delta declines markedly, and at about age 3 years there is predominately diffuse theta with less frequent delta waves. Between ages 3 and 6 years, diffuse theta declines further, paralleling the increase in the posterior dominant rhythm. By age 8 years some theta persists, as it does for the next few years. This is where confusion arises. We find a wide range of theta prominence in young subjects with no demonstrable cerebral pathology on imaging studies and no neurological deficits. Thus, unless there is some clinical correlation for "excessive" slowing, particularly in the theta range, it is best to be generous in determining whether or not there is too much theta. On the other hand, if there is a great deal of delta after age 4 or 5 years, the odds are that there indeed is cerebral dysfunction. Observe that diffuse slowing, regardless of degree, must be symmetrical.

**Note**: It is particularly important to obtain a true waking record in children. They frequently are drowsy, or rapidly become so. Thus, assessment of slowing must be made during the alert state. Technicians have a tendency to let a drowsy child fall asleep, and this is fine. But, after obtaining a sufficient drowsy or sleeping record, the child should be aroused in order to determine the nature of the waking background.

Hyperventilation (HV) is an important procedure in children (see section on HV). It may come as a surprise that a young child can be taught to hyperventilate quite well. The trick is to make the task interesting. One solution is to employ a "hyperventilation toy," a device developed some years ago by colleagues of one of the authors (C.D. Binnie and T. Wisman). Such a device can be made easily by someone in your bioengineering department or even by you. The principle is transduction of the exhaled breath (blowing) to an electric current. An example might be a small bear with small light-bulbs for eyes and a large colored button on his tummy. As the child blows on the button the eyes light up, much to the child's delight. There are many possible variations on this theme, but the principle is the same. A marked build-up of generalized high-voltage delta activity is the usual response. If this does not occur, it probably is due to inadequate hyperventilation.

Photic stimulation is an important procedure in children with epilepsy, and care must be taken because of an increased number of subjects with photosensitivity (e.g. a photoparoxysmal or photoconvulsive response consisting of generalized polyspike-wave discharges) as compared with adults. This is due primarily to a higher incidence of active primary generalized epilepsy in the young (see section on activation procedures).

With respect to sleep, some characteristics in children differ from those in adults. In particular, at about age 1 year and continuing for several years, drowsiness (Stage I sleep) elicits a response known by a rather intimidating term – hypnagogic hypersynchrony (A-18). The response consists of paroxysmal, synchronous, high-voltage, rhythmic 4 to 5 Hz waves in diffuse distribution. These waves occur in runs lasting from a few to several seconds, and are unassociated with epileptiform activity such as spike discharges. The response is quite dramatic in some subjects but is entirely normal. The response usually declines by age 5 or 6 years.

As the child enters Stage II sleep the synchronous waves are replaced by diffuse slowing in both theta and delta ranges. The background voltage tends to be higher than in older subjects. Sleep spindles may be most prominent in the frontal regions, particularly in young children, and high-voltage spindles are not uncommon. Important to note is the evolution of spindle synchrony. Sleep spindles are usually present at birth, but over the next five to six months they occur asynchronously, alternating from side to side. By six months, spindle synchrony is usually present in most infants (A-16, A-17).

Unlike adults, children often descend into SWS with diffuse often very high-voltage delta activity. As in adults, sleep spindles decline during this stage. Note that SWS sometimes dominates the entire recording if the child has been sedated. Unfortunately, this circumstance may obscure focal abnormalities and even frank epileptiform activity in some children.

## SPECIAL CONSIDERATIONS IN THE ELDERLY

The elderly present particular challenges in EEG interpretation. We realize that any generalization is open to exceptions. Nonetheless, certain aspects of recording in the aged and interpretation of the resultant record deserve mention.

As is evident in any large EEG department, the number of requests for older patients has increased over the years. At this time, about 40 percent of our requests are for individuals older than 60 years. Such patients are often quite ill, many with multisystem disease. Many are confused. In fact, the most common reasons for requests in the elderly are "altered mental status," "syncope," or loss of consciousness of unknown cause. Not infrequently the cause turns out to be seizures, principally complex partial in type. In particular, non-convulsive status epilepticus may be discovered. Other common reasons for referral are dementia, stroke, and metabolic derangement.

At the outset let us stipulate that the EEG in the elderly, regardless of age, can be normal in every regard. This extends to the alpha rhythm, which, in rare cases, may maintain a steady 10 Hz frequency throughout life (A-6). The authors recently saw the record of a centenarian who had beautifully organized 10 Hz alpha! The usual progression, however, is a gradual decline in the frequency of the posterior dominant rhythm. A specific disease process may not be evident, but the slower PDR probably reflects a degree of cerebral dysfunction (e.g. cerebral vascular disease or a degenerative process). Another common finding is intermittent bitemporal delta activity, symmetric or asymmetric, perhaps preponderant on one side. Although the delta waves probably represent underlying cerebral pathology, for example some degree of cerebrovascular disease, there may be no focal abnormality on an imaging study. We emphasize this because the ordering clinician should be aware that such a patient is relatively unlikely to have a brain tumor or stroke.

The elderly tend to develop more bifrontal delta activity during drowsiness than younger subjects. In common with bitemporal delta, this feature may have no specific significance. It is likely that the bifrontal delta may represent some degree of subcortical dysfunction secondary to vascular disease or other degenerative factors. It is not, however, particularly helpful in making a specific diagnosis.

Sleep features in the elderly tend to be less well defined than those encountered in younger adults. Sleep spindles may be more irregular or of lower voltage. Similarly, vertex sharp waves may be less well defined. A great deal of diffuse slowing is common, even in earlier stages of sleep. Again, such findings are of limited diagnostic utility.

A word about recording the EEG in older subjects is in order. The elderly often find it difficult to relax. Muscle and movement artifact may be prominent, and chewing artifact is not uncommon. Despite the technician's best efforts the artifacts may persist. It is the job of the electroencephalographer to make the best of the situation. There are usually a few interpretable segments, even in the most artifact-ridden record, that allow some statement on the nature of background activities. Discovering epileptiform activity may be difficult if not impossible, but a hunt for discharges hiding within the artifact sometimes pays dividends. If necessary, a repeat EEG after mild sedation may be indicated. This recommendation depends on the clinical circumstances and whether the ordering clinician truly requires additional EEG data.

## ACTIVATION PROCEDURES

### Hyperventilation

Hyperventilation (HV) is a standard procedure during routine EEG recording. It is easily carried out, though the technician must be instructed on the proper method. The usefulness of HV depends on vasoconstriction secondary to resultant decreased $CO_2$ concentration, thus inducing relative cerebral ischemia and decreased glucose utilization. Subjects may complain of lightheadedness or tingling in the extremities. Even tetany secondary to hypocalcemia may occur with particularly vigorous HV. The procedure is most effective in the young; in the elderly it has little effect.

Latent abnormalities may be brought out during HV, and new abnormalities may be produced. These include epileptiform discharges and focal slowing (see discussion below). The standard response is moderate to high-voltage delta activity with distinct bifrontal preponderance (A-19). The delta is usually rhythmic and occurs in repeated runs. In the young, nearly continuous delta may be evoked. As a rule, HV is carried out for 3 minutes with vigorous exhalation at an increased but not particularly rapid rate. Rapid HV moves little air and has correspondingly little effect. After the conclusion of HV the record should return to baseline levels in about 1 minute. If return to baseline occurs after a protracted period, it may represent an abnormality. The classical cause of a long return to baseline is hypoglycemia.

HV is often omitted in subjects over the age of 65 years due to its low yield. An elderly person's vascular system, probably due to disease, is less responsive to the metabolic changes precipitated by HV. In cases of suspected epilepsy, however, HV may be useful despite these limitations. Note that there are few contraindications for performing HV. Perhaps the most important are pulmonary and cardiac disease. HV may be performed in patients with brain tumors although, if the resting record reveals clear focal slowing, the procedure probably offers little additional information.

**Intermittent Photic Stimulation**

Intermittent photic stimulation (IPS) is another standard procedure during routine EEG recording. The procedure is easily carried out with modern strobe units linked to computer programs. IPS evokes a rhythmic frequency in the occipital derivations termed the "following response." The response is also known as the "driving response," though the former term is preferred. If the response to the flash train is 1:1 it is termed the fundamental. It is not unusual to see harmonic (twice the flash frequency, A-20) and/or subharmonic (half the flash frequency) responses.

The frequency range of the evoked waves varies greatly, and there may be no response at all. The latter has no pathological significance. The response is sometimes quite prominent at low flash frequencies, say 1 per second. This is termed the "on" response and in fact represents a visual evoked response. If the following response is absent on one side, it may support a diagnosis of unilateral structural disease involving the occipital region (e.g. infarction in posterior cerebral artery territory). If a patient is demented and agitated, resulting in a great deal of artifact, IPS should be omitted inasmuch as it is useless. The major utility of the procedure is in patients with epilepsy suspected of having seizures precipitated by flickering light. There are various degrees of photosensitivity, the most prominent being a synchronous high-voltage spike/polyspike wave discharge (photoparoxysmal response; also known as the photoconvulsive response; see section on EEG in epilepsy). Photosensitivity is often maximal at 14 to 16 flashes per second. Some patients demonstrate a photoparoxysmal response at a specific frequency, or a very narrow frequency band. For patients with a marked degree of photosensitivity, an abnormal response may be obtained over a wide frequency range.

There are lesser degrees of photosensitivity. For example, one may see occipital spikes that are time-linked to the flash train. In this case, the spikes cease when the strobe is stopped.

Note that the technician must stop the flash train if generalized polyspike-wave bursts occur. If the stimulus is continued, a generalized convulsion may result. Typically, the evoked discharges outlast cessation of the flash stimulus by a second or so.

## Sleep Deprivation

Sleep deprivation is a powerful activator of epileptiform activity. It is the procedure of choice in patients with suspected epilepsy who either have normal routine EEGs, or minor suggestive findings during routine recording (e.g. a few ill-defined sharp waves). It is often suggested that the subject stay up all night before his or her appointment the next morning, but a brief period of sleep may be permitted. In the latter case the patient is instructed to stay up late, sleep for 1 or 2 hours, and then come to the EEG laboratory for testing in the morning. No stimulants such as coffee, tea, or colas are permitted. The recording should be 1 hour in duration. Hyperventilation is carried out early in the test, after which the patient is allowed to sleep. One can expect an increase in or *de novo* appearance of focal epileptiform activity in about 30 percent of patients with epilepsy. It should be noted that sleep deprivation in and of itself is activating. In other words, it is not absolutely necessary for the patient to sleep during the test in order to obtain positive results.

## Sedated Sleep

Sedated sleep is an effective activation procedure and is most often carried out in children. It is also useful in adults who are restless, or in patients with dementia who pose difficulties because of excessive movement. A useful agent to promote sleep is chloral hydrate. This has a relatively rapid onset of action and results in little hangover, and it also has a broad therapeutic index. In general it is better to administer a larger rather than a smaller dose in order to avoid successive administration of the drug. Of note is that chloral hydrate produces a great deal of beta activity, often of high voltage. This feature may be confounding, especially in children who may slip into SWS, thus producing a marked beta/delta record that obscures focal findings.

# NORMAL VARIANTS AND PAROXYSMAL PHENOMENA OF UNCERTAIN SIGNIFICANCE

## Alpha Variants

Slow alpha variant appears in the occipital regions at a frequency one-half that of the ongoing alpha (A-9). Suspect its presence when posterior rhythmic theta activity has a notched appearance, revealing its subharmonic relationship to the alpha. Tabulation of the notch frequency shows it to be twice the theta frequency. Slow alpha variant has the same characteristics as alpha itself – for example, it attenuates with eye opening. Fast alpha variant also appears in the occipital areas and has a frequency twice that of the alpha (A-8). These variants may alternate with the alpha, or the alpha may not be present at all. Both are normal.

## Rhythmic mid-temporal theta discharges (RMTD)

This was formerly known as psychomotor variant. Rhythmic sharply con-toured theta waves at 5 to 6 Hz appearing in the mid-temporal regions (A-21). The bursts are brief, usually 1 sec or so in duration, and may be unilateral or independent in both mid-temporal regions. At times, one of the waves may stand out from the others, giving the appearance of a sharp wave. Noting the durations of the waveforms to be similar, regardless of variations in amplitude, makes the diagnosis. This phenomenon appears during drowsiness and has no clear clinical significance. Incidentally, psychomotor variant (the old term) was meant to suggest that this phenomenon might be correlated with complex partial seizures (formerly psychomotor seizures). In fact, this usually does not turn out to be the case. Nonetheless, RMTD is sometimes considered an abnormality by the inexperienced.

## Wicket Spikes

Sharply contoured rhythmic frequency varying from 7 to 11 Hz, maximal in the mid-temporal derivations, occurring in brief runs. Wicket spikes are differ-entiated from RMTD by waveform and frequency. This finding occurs during drowsiness and has no apparent clinical significance. The reader should compare the locations of wicket spikes and mu rhythm [the latter is found in the central (Rolandic) regions].

## Subclinical Rhythmical Electroencephalographic Discharges of Adults (SREDA)

SREDA masquerades as an ictal discharge in one or both temporal regions. For the unwary, SREDA appears to be an electrographic seizure. The discharge appears during wakefulness, arises suddenly from a normal background, and has a duration of several seconds. The rhythmic waveform is in the theta range with admixed fast components. There are no clear-cut spikes and no recruitment (an ictal discharge consisting of the sudden onset of rapid low-voltage waves, gradually declining in frequency and increasing in amplitude; A-46, A-47). Moreover, the patient has no alteration of awareness and is fully responsive. SREDA has no known significance beyond the fact that it must be recognized as non-epileptiform in order to avoid misdiagnosis.

## Small Sharp Spikes

Small sharp spikes (SSS) are low-amplitude, rapid spikes. They appear in both hemispheres as synchronous or asynchronous events, most often in the temporal derivations, and become evident during drowsiness and light sleep. They are not thought to be associated with epilepsy. Small sharp spikes are also known as benign epileptiform transients of sleep (BETS).

## Phantom Spike-Wave Discharges

Phantom spike-waves are low-voltage, usually synchronous discharges at a frequency of 6 Hz appearing symmetrically in the parieto-posterior temporal derivations. The spike itself is usually less prominent than the following slow wave. They appear individually or in brief rhythmic runs and do not have known epileptogenic significance.

## 14 and 6 (14/6) Positive Spikes

14 and 6 positive spikes, as the name implies, are positive in polarity. They are usually maximal in the posterior quadrants and appear in isolation or in groups. They may be unilateral or bilateral. The two frequencies are often admixed, but one may predominate. The phenomenon appears during drowsiness and is best recorded with crossed ear references (essentially wide interelectrode distances). In the past, 14/6 was thought to be associated with a wide variety of conditions including psychiatric disorders and epilepsy. Although there remains some disagreement as to their significance, they have no known relationship to epilepsy.

# 3

# THE ABNORMAL EEG

## NON-EPILEPTIFORM ABNORMAL PATTERNS

### Focal Slowing

As we have seen, slow waves in and of themselves are not abnormal, but slowing that is localized or lateralized commands our attention. In fact, the EEG is highly sensitive to the presence of localized cerebral pathology, in some cases more so than imaging studies. The most important focal abnormality is delta activity (0.5–3.5 Hz) occurring in any cerebral location. Focal delta waves are a good indicator of structural disease, which means any lesion, usually (but not always) demonstrable on imaging studies, that disrupts cerebral architecture. At times, and especially in the elderly, focal temporal delta may not correlate with an evident structural lesion on MRI/CT studies, even though cerebral pathology of some degree underlies the EEG finding.

Processes producing focal delta include brain tumors, cerebral infarction, brain abscess, subdural hematoma, intracerebral hemorrhage, and other traumatic brain injuries. Focal rhythmic and arrhythmic delta activity also occurs following focal seizures and may accompany focal interictal activity. Delta foci are often most evident in the temporal derivations, even when the main pathology is not in the temporal lobe. We term this *false localization*, the slowing being projected to the temporal regions from deeper or adjacent structures. Determining the site of a delta focus is precisely the same as determining the site of focal spiking.

Brain tumors represent the prototype of a process producing focal slowing (A-59a, 59b). The type and extent of the slowing depends on tumor type, rapidity of growth, and location. Malignant, rapidly growing tumors (e.g. glioblastoma and metastatic tumors) produce irregular, polymorphic delta activity (polymorphic in the sense of varying waveform and frequency). Note that associated theta frequencies may be present, and beta activity may be depressed over the involved area. Voltage is variable but is generally moderate. Polymorphic delta is thought to be generated from lesions involving the white matter. Contrast this with rhythmic delta activity that results from lesions of gray matter – either cortex or subcortical nuclear sites (e.g. thalamus). It should be clear, therefore, that polymorphic and rhythmic delta may coexist when lesions involves both cortex and subcortical white matter. (For another type of rhythmic delta that is bifrontal in location, see section on projected rhythms.)

Associated spike or sharp wave discharges are not common in rapidly growing tumors, even though the patient may present with seizures. A slowly growing low-grade astrocytoma also produces focal delta activity that, overall, is less prominent than in the case of malignant tumors. Theta activity may be more prominent than delta. The slower-growing tumors are more likely to be associated with epileptiform activity than malignant processes. It should be noted that very slowly growing infiltrating gliomas may produce little (if any) slowing until they become relatively large. A good example is the low-grade astrocytoma of childhood that presents as recurrent seizures. In such cases there may be epileptiform activity in the involved location with little focal slowing.

The meningioma is the prototype of a slowly expanding tumor that is likely to produce a theta focus (4–7 Hz). It should be noted, however, that the EEG may be normal in some cases. Accompanying spike/sharp wave discharges are not uncommon. If the process begins to invaginate the cerebral cortex, perhaps indicating more rapid growth or more gradual displacement of intracranial contents, more prominent slowing is recorded including delta waves.

Intraventricular tumors, for example those within the lateral ventricles, sometimes result in a slow wave focus in the adjacent temporal region – a false localizing feature. Tumors of the third ventricle do not ordinarily result in focal slowing; rather, projected rhythmic delta activity to the frontal derivations is likely (see section on projected rhythms).

Mention should be made of brain abscesses. While relatively uncommon nowadays, the brain abscess is said to produce the most prominent and slowest polymorphic delta focus with destruction of other cortical rhythms. This is true earlier on in the development of the abscess when there is a great deal of associated edema. When the abscess is chronic and encapsulated, however, focal slowing is much less prominent.

In summary, the reader should be aware that slowly growing tumors or other focal processes produce much less slowing than rapidly developing lesions. When growth is very gradual the EEG may be normal. Epileptiform discharges are more common in slowly developing lesions than those that grow rapidly.

## Diffuse Slowing

The presence of diffuse slowing suggests bilateral cerebral dysfunction with a broad spectrum of causes. The first major problem in making a determination of diffuse slowing is the patient's state of alertness. Many patients are quite drowsy throughout EEG recording. This, of course, produces slowing of the record and would not necessarily be abnormal. The electroencephalographer must diagnose the presence of diffuse slowing during the most alert segments of recording. If this is not possible, one may have to say that the diffuse slowing may be in part, if not wholly, due to drowsiness, although a degree of cerebral pathology cannot be excluded.

A second problem relates to medication. We encounter this frequently, especially with referrals from psychiatry. Many psychotropic drugs cause diffuse slowing (see section on effects of drugs on the EEG). Not only this, but the posterior dominant rhythm may be slowed as well. While it is true that the record is abnormal in such cases, the patient may demonstrate no obvious neurological dysfunction. Thus, when reporting this abnormality, it is important to state that the background slowing is likely due to an effect of medication(s) that the patient is taking.

Many pathological processes lead to diffuse slowing as well as slowing of the PDR. Alzheimer's disease, multi-infarct dementia, various toxic-metabolic disorders, post-ictal states, and congenital brain damage come to mind. The reader is referred to individual sections dealing with these conditions.

## Projected Rhythms

Projected rhythmic activity, usually in the delta range, is also known as "rhythm at a distance." This important EEG finding is indicative of a process that involves deep midline structures, that is, a compromise of peri-third ventricular structures (thalamus), either directly or indirectly. The prototype of projected rhythms is frontal intermittent rhythmic delta activity (FIRDA). FIRDA, as the name implies, is a rhythmic, usually high-voltage delta frequency at 2 to 3 Hz that predominates in the frontal regions (A-55). Occasionally, higher or lower frequencies are recorded. It is usually discontinuous and must be differentiated from repetitive eye blink artifact. The two often coexist. A differential point is posterior extension of the potential field in the case of FIRDA, while eye blink artifact is usually confined to the frontal regions. Most laboratories employ two periorbital electrodes (e.g. at the superior and lateral aspects of the orbit) to aid in recognition of eye movement artifact.

A variety of pathological processes result in FIRDA including tumors, increased intracranial pressure (ICP) of any cause, and toxic-metabolic disorders. A good example of the value of FIRDA is in the diagnosis of a frontal lobe tumor. The expanding lesion begins to compromise the deep midline as well as frontal cortical and subcortical tissue. The combination produces focal polymorphic frontal delta activity with associated FIRDA. In these cases the FIRDA may be asymmetric, the higher voltage occurring on the side of the lesion. Such patients may present with headache, personality changes, and seizures prompting both EEG and imaging studies.

FIRDA is a classical finding in increased ICP of whatever cause. In general, FIRDA is most prominent if ICP is relatively acute. When ICP is chronic, however, FIRDA is less evident or even absent. Metabolic disorders (e.g. electrolyte imbalance or uremia) may also result in FIRDA, even though there is no evidence of ICP. In these cases the deep midline structures are affected by the generalized cerebral dysfunction.

There are other examples of projected rhythms. Occipital intermittent rhythmic delta activity (OIRDA) results from an occipital lesion impinging on the posterior third ventricle. Likewise, temporal intermittent rhythmic delta activity (TIRDA) is recorded in deep temporal lesions affecting a lateral ventricle. Both these rhythms appear in the 2 to 3 Hz band and are usually, as the name implies, intermittent. As with FIRDA, they may coexist with irregular slowing in the area of interest due to both cortical and subcortical involvement.

## Periodicity

This EEG term refers to a periodic pattern consisting of discharges of various forms occurring at more or less fixed intervals, often followed by suppression of cerebral activity. In fact, inasmuch as true periodicity is uncommon, some prefer the term pseudoperiodicity. Periodic discharges are indicative of significant cerebral disease, whether focal or generalized.

### *Periodic Lateralized Epileptiform Discharges (PLEDs)*

This entity is a well-known example of periodicity. PLEDs denote focal lesions and have been described most frequently in acute infarcts. They have also been found in malignant neoplastic lesions, brain abscess, and encephalitis (A-51, A-52). Note that PLEDs are usually not associated with slowly growing lesions. (In the early description of PLEDs, associated metabolic abnormality was mentioned as a contributing cause.)

Herpes simplex encephalitis is an infrequent but important cause of PLEDs. In this condition the periodic discharges consist of high-voltage sharp potentials over one or even both temporal lobes, occurring every few seconds. In cases of suspected meningoencephalitis with perhaps inconclusive imaging or cerebrospinal fluid studies, the finding of periodicity in a temporal region can lead to early antiviral treatment.

In cerebral infarction, PLEDs are usually recorded in a location adjacent to the acute infarct, presumably due to the relative unreactivity of the severely damaged cortex. The adjacent cortex is only partially affected by the pathological process and appears capable of generating the discharges. PLEDs are characterized by repetitive discharges, usually stereotyped, consisting of high-voltage sharp waves with or without associated slow components. In general they are continual. The period varies, but the discharges usually occur every 1 to 2 seconds.

A fundamental question raised by PLEDs is that of their potential epileptogenicity – that is, do they imply that the patient is likely to develop seizures? The answer is mixed. Many patients do indeed develop seizures, apparently resulting from the PLEDs, but some do not. In several patients the authors have recorded PLEDs that evolved into clear electrographic seizures with clear-cut recruiting rhythms (without obvious change in the patient's mental status). As the electrographic seizures subsided, the PLED patterns were restored. In other cases such patients develop clinical seizures that originate from the involved hemisphere. In still others no clinical or electrographic seizures result. This variability leaves open the question of treating patients with PLEDs. Some experts treat PLEDs with antiepileptic drugs (e.g. loading the patient with phenytoin), even if there is no obvious clinical seizure activity. Another reason for treating without clinical seizures is the concept that the ongoing discharges interrupt cortical function, for example a patient with a dominant hemispheric lesion characterized by aphasia. The authors have treated such individuals with mixed results. We believe that one should not be overly aggressive in an attempt to suppress PLEDs. On the other hand, if the patient has clear clinical or electrographic seizures, treatment is clearly indicated. A final note: PLEDs are self limited, usually resolving over several days time.

### Periodic Epileptiform Discharges (PEDs)

These discharges are generalized, recurring with periods of one or a few seconds. The discharges vary in waveform but are usually characterized by synchronous high-voltage spikes or sharp waves. PEDs are indicative of generalized convulsive status epilepticus of the subtle type (see section on status epilepticus). They arise after a period of overt generalized status and are associated with coma along with minor motor manifestations. PEDs are also seen as a result of cerebral anoxia secondary to cardiopulmonary arrest – also thought to be indicative of subtle status. Note that, in the absence of historical data, PEDs as described above resemble certain types of discharges found in non-convulsive status epilepticus (see section on this topic).

### Subacute sclerosing panencephalitis (SSPE)

Fortunately, we rarely encounter patients with this terrible disease, thanks to widespread vaccination against the measles virus. The condition was not unusual in the past, but in the United States today there are perhaps two to three cases per annum. The patient usually presents with recurrent myoclonic jerks. At onset there may be no other neurological or cognitive findings. The EEG demonstrates periodic discharges consisting of generalized multiphasic high-voltage slow waves, often with associated sharp components (A-53). The period is relatively long, approximately 5 to 8 seconds. Each discharge is associated with a myoclonic jerk that may be either rapid or relatively slow. The background may be preserved at first, but gradually deteriorates. In late stages the periodic discharges remain, followed by a low-voltage featureless background. Eventually the discharges disappear. At this point the patient is severely impaired, and death soon follows.

### Creutzfeld-Jakob disease (CJD)

The discharges in CJD are distinctive, as is their periodicity. They commonly consist of low- to moderate-amplitude biphasic sharp waves with a period of 700 to 900 ms (A-63). At first, the discharges may be sporadic, even focal, and minor, multifocal myoclonic jerks may be observed. Eventually the sharp waves become generalized, associated with generalized synchronous myoclonic jerks. The discharges disappear before death, and the background rhythms are destroyed, leaving a marked and diffuse depression of cerebral activity. (See also the section on dementia.)

### Burst-Suppression

The term burst-suppression refers to a cycling of marked depression of cerebral activity and bursts of cerebral activity of variable amplitude, duration, and waveform. The bursts may be comprised of multiphasic delta components, admixtures of various frequencies, or epileptiform activity such as spikes or sharp waves, often with admixed slow components (A-54). The prototype of this phenomenon is found in patients receiving general anesthesia. It is thought that burst-suppression results from suppression of cortical activity via GABA-ergic mechanisms with breakthrough of EEG activity due to intact glutaminergic transmission. Under progressively deepening anesthesia there are progressive EEG changes ranging from normal sleep patterns, diffuse delta waves, burst-suppression, and isopotentiality.

Burst-suppression also occurs in patients with cardiopulmonary arrest who suffer from cerebral anoxia, and after severe head injuries. In both cases the prognosis is poor. Another setting is the period following overt generalized convulsive status-epilepticus (GCSE) in which the prognosis is better. In patients with GCSE of the subtle type, however, a burst-suppression pattern implies a poor prognosis, especially if the bursts contain spikes or sharp waves. Resolution of status depends on eradication of all epileptiform activity. Burst-suppression may be encountered in neonates, usually those with severe cerebral damage or certain rare syndromes. The prognosis in such cases is usually poor.

## EPILEPTIFORM PATTERNS

The EEG finds its most important application in epilepsy. With the advent of imaging (both CT and MRI), the EEG's previous important role in diagnosing brain tumors has virtually disappeared. In epilepsy, however, the test continues to be an important mainstay in diagnosis, follow-up and, to some extent, prognosis. Despite the important role of the EEG, the diagnosis of epilepsy in most instances rests on clinical grounds. Epileptiform EEGs can be recorded in persons without epilepsy. Likewise, patients with epilepsy not infrequently have no such discharges in routine recording. Nonetheless, the EEG can provide important supporting evidence for a diagnosis of epilepsy. Moreover, the type of epilepsy may be confirmed, or actually diagnosed. For example, the EEG differentiates between localization-related and generalized epilepsies, and is a principal feature in the definition of epilepsy syndromes.

Note that a strict definition of epileptiform discharges is confined to spikes and spike-wave complexes, and of course electrographic ictal discharges. In reality, other paroxysmal patterns have similar significance, for example sharp waves. The following paragraphs provide direction concerning specific findings in epilepsy.

## The Spike

The spike is defined as paroxysmal potential (i.e. it arises suddenly from the background) that is very sharp in contour (you can prick your finger on it), and whose rise has a steeper slope than that of its decline. Its duration is 20 to 80 ms thus differentiating it from more rapid muscle action potentials. Spikes are usually electronegative at the surface, although there are exceptions. The spike is usually followed by a low-voltage slow potential (duration of about 200 ms) before the baseline is re-established. In some cases the slow wave may not be evident. Spikes may occur in isolation, in groups of two or more (A-45), or in repetitive runs. They may be focal, multifocal or generalized.

## The Spike-Wave Complex

The spike-wave complex consists of two components – the spike and the accompanying time-locked slow wave. The prototype is the generalized spike-wave complex recorded in patients with simple absence attacks as a manifestation of primary generalized epilepsy (PGE) (A-42, A-43). In this case the complex is in the 3 (± 0.5) Hz frequency band. The discharge is relatively high in voltage (say 200–300 µV or more), and the slow wave usually higher in amplitude than the spike. Both the spike and wave are surface negative, and the discharge may be focal or generalized. Note that generalized polyspike-wave complexes also may be recorded in patients with PGE (A-44).

Spike-wave complexes also occur at frequencies other than 3 Hz. The generalized, slow spike-wave complex (sometimes known as petit mal variant) is in reality a sharp-slow complex in the 2 Hz frequency band. The prototype occurs in Lennox–Gastaut syndrome (LGS) and is generalized with bifrontal preponderance. Rapid generalized spike-wave complexes occur in patients with primary generalized epilepsy, especially those with generalized tonic-clonic convulsions. In these cases the frequency band is typically about 5 Hz. Another distinctive pattern is the generalized irregular polyspike-wave discharge at 6 to 8 Hz, characteristic of juvenile myoclonic epilepsy (JME).

## The Sharp Wave

Although sharp waves do not fall into the strict definition of epileptiform activity (spikes and spike-wave complexes), for all practical purposes they have a similar significance when recorded in patients with epilepsy. The sharp wave is defined as a paroxysmal sharp potential (not as sharp as a spike) that has a duration of 80 to 200 ms. As with the spike discharge, the upswing of the sharp wave should be steeper than the downswing. A following relatively low-voltage slow wave is not uncommon. When focal, the sharp wave is thought to be less localizing than the spike, probably because it is generated by a more extensive neuronal network than the spike.

## Other Interictal Paroxysmal Waveforms

Other paroxysmal potentials are seen in patients with epilepsy, although they are less specific than the above features. A few examples will suffice to make the point. Patients with long-standing epilepsy and generalized seizures, possibly in remission, commonly have generalized irregular slow-wave discharges, sometimes with included sharp components. Patients with treated simple absence attacks may demonstrate brief rhythmic high-voltage 3 Hz slow-wave discharges without accompanying spikes. Such discharges probably represent the remnants of previous 3 Hz spike-wave activity. Another relatively non-specific discharge sometimes encountered in patients with partial epilepsy is the focal theta or even delta discharge. The slow waves may or may not demonstrate a sharp contour. They are, however, paroxysmal (standing out from the background) and give a clue to the location of the epileptogenic focus. Such findings are definitely not epileptiform *per se*. In such cases, when the EEG is performed for diagnostic purposes, a follow-up activation EEG (sleep deprivation) is indicated in an attempt to record clear-cut epileptiform activity.

Epileptiform discharges are sometimes recorded in persons without epilepsy. Thus, spikes themselves do not make the diagnosis. A small proportion of normal individuals may have a few spikes in the EEG. These discharges do not imply that the person will develop seizures. Similar considerations apply to relatives of patients with PGE. The generalized 3 Hz spike-wave complex is considered by some to be an inherited characteristic as, of course, is PGE itself. Such individuals may demonstrate spike-wave complexes in the EEG without ever developing clinical seizures. This emphasizes the futility of making a diagnosis of epilepsy on the basis of the EEG alone. (It should be mentioned, however, that brief bursts of synchronous spike-wave complexes can be associated with a decline in reaction time, determined by specific testing. This finding, of course, would indicate the patient has brief impairment of cerebral function despite the lack of a positive clinical history.)

Another example of spike or sharp wave discharges in persons without epilepsy is migraine. Although the results of studies vary, two sorts of discharges may be recorded. Spike or sharp wave discharges in the temporal regions have been described in some patients with classical migraine. In those with so-called complicated migraine, spike-wave discharges have been recorded. This raises the question of the relationship of migraine to epilepsy. This brief book is not the forum for discussion of this issue, which is controversial. Suffice it to say that the two conditions sometimes coexist but, overall, there is limited evidence for a direct linkage.

## Location and Significance of Focal Epileptiform Discharges

### Temporal spikes

The most common sites for focal epileptiform activity are the temporal lobes (A-39, A-40). In patients with complex partial epilepsy the discharges may be maximum in the anterior temporal regions at the F7and/or the F8 electrodes (the F7/8 electrodes also record spikes originating from the inferior frontal cortex). Note, however, that discharges in these cases may demonstrate a focal maximum between the anterior and mid-temporal electrodes (F7-T3 or F8-T4), or indeed at the mid-temporal electrodes (T3/4). (Some laboratories employ T1 and T2 electrodes, placed inferior to F7/8. The temporal lobe spike may be more evident and of higher amplitude at these locations.)

Discharges may be infrequent, even rare – or they may be frequent. The frequency of recorded discharges, however, has a weak correlation with the patient's seizure control, although it is true that the number of discharges tends to decline in persistently seizure-free patients.

In patients with complex partial epilepsy the underlying pathology often resides in the hippocampus, commonly originating in infancy. Prolonged febrile convulsions are a potential cause, as are birth trauma, prolonged labor, and early hypoxia. A warning or aura – a common type being the rising epigastric sensation (RES) – often heralds the clinically observable seizures. Alternatively, the patient may report a feeling of fear or an unpleasant olfactory sensation. These symptoms originate within the deep anterior temporal structures and, in fact, are simple partial seizures. The surface EEG usually does not display epileptiform activity during this phase of the seizure. Recording during EEG monitoring with placement of depth electrodes displays the seizure onset before any surface manifestations are evident.

If spikes are independent in the temporal lobes, it is difficult to determine, on grounds of the EEG, which temporal lobe generates the clinical seizure activity. The more active focus may not be responsible for the patient's recurrent seizures as has been shown with intensive EEG-video monitoring. Alternatively, the seizures may emanate from either temporal lobe at various times. Thus, when rendering the EEG report, one may say that the patient's seizures are likely to originate from one or both temporal lobes.

Mid-temporal spikes may have a different significance from the foregoing. Such discharges are seen after significant head trauma or with a temporal lobe tumor, resulting in damage to the temporal cortex. Of interest is that the much discussed auras of déjà vu, jamai vu, and formed visual hallucinations are generally associated with lesions of the temporal cortex, not the deep anterior temporal structures.

Note that the posterior temporal spike (T5/T6) usually results from more posterior temporal cortical damage and may result from infarction or other pathology in the region of the posterior cerebral circulation.

### Occipital spikes

The occipital spike focus (O1/O2) is distinctive and usually found in children with occipital epilepsy (see section on epilepsy syndromes). Care must be taken in discovering its existence, for it is easy to concentrate on other brain areas, particularly the temporal regions, and neglect the occipital regions save for determining the frequency of the PDR. This is especially true when the spikes are infrequent, for they are easily obscured by ongoing background activity. One method of assessing possible occipital spikes is to record for a period with the patient's eyes open. Important to note is the downward deviation of the spike in the occipital channels during bipolar A-P recording (double banana). There is no phase-reversal because the occipital electrode is the last in the chain. Were one to place electrodes beneath O1/O2 (suboccipital), the phase reversal would become apparent.

An electrode arrangement (montage) that is useful in recording occipital events is referred to as the circle or headband bipolar arrangement. Here, the electrodes are linked around the scalp, running through the occipital and frontopolar electrodes. Thus, any occipital spike will demonstrate a phase reversal at O1 or O2 (A-41a). Referential recording, on the other hand, simply demonstrates the highest amplitude at the occipital electrode (A-41b). Note also that an occipital spike focus may be manifest in both occipital regions, the side of higher amplitude being the putative focus.

The clinical history may help in directing attention to the occipital regions inasmuch as such patients often report visual symptoms consisting of bright or flashing lights, or a grid pattern (not formed visual hallucinations such as scenes or persons). The latter occur in patients with complex partial seizures of temporal cortical origin. Also, some patients experience complex partial seizures resulting from anterior spread of the ictal discharge. The EEG diagnosis is important in that occipital epilepsy presenting in childhood usually has a favorable prognosis, both for immediate seizure control and eventual seizure subsidence. The same may not apply to adults.

### Centro-temporal spikes

These spikes are also distinctive, and once seen are not forgotten. They are the accompaniment of benign epilepsy of childhood with centrotemporal spikes (BECTS) – formerly Rolandic epilepsy. The discharges are clearly focal at the central (C3/4) electrodes with representation at the mid-temporal (T4/C4) electrodes. They usually consist of biphasic spikes of variable amplitude and are markedly activated during drowsiness and sleep. In fact, they may only be evident when the patient is drowsy or asleep. The spikes occur in isolation or sometimes in rhythmic runs or groups. They may be unilateral or, most commonly, bilaterally independent. The background rhythms are normal during wakefulness and sleep. During sleep, care must be taken to differentiate the spikes from ongoing vertex activity, especially if the latter is very prominent and sharp. The broader distribution of the potential field of centro-temporal spikes as well as their independent occurrence in the two hemispheres should give sufficient clues to their recognition. The waveform may also be a differential point, although this is not always reliable.

### Frontal and fronto-polar spikes

These discharges are recorded in patients with seizures originating in the frontal lobes. The fronto-polar spike (Fp1/Fp2) is thought to be generated by orbital frontal cortex or adjacent areas, whereas the frontal spike at the mid-frontal electrode(s) (F3/F4) is generated by the frontal convexity. The fronto-polar spike when recorded on an A-P bipolar arrangement is an up-going potential in channels Fp1/2–F7/8 and Fp1/2–F3/4. As in the case of occipital spikes there is no phase reversal (Fp1/2 are the first electrodes in the chain). These discharges are well displayed with the bipolar circle (hatband) montage. A problem with identifying frontal spikes (or sharp waves) is eye-blink artifact, especially if frequent. Usually eyeblinks are symmetrical in the two hemispheres, whereas fronto-polar spikes are likely to be lateralized. Some recording should be carried out with the patient holding his or her eyes gently closed with mild downward pressure on the globes. As with occipital spikes, there may be representation in the opposite hemisphere at lower voltage, presumably due either to spread of the potential field, or to transcallosal transmission.

Focal frontal spikes sometimes precede a generalized spike-wave discharge. This is termed *secondary bilateral synchrony* and is the electrographic equivalent of secondarily generalized seizures. In this case the spike-wave complexes are usually irregular, in contrast to the 3 per second spike-wave discharges of simple absence attacks. Care must be taken to determine whether there is a consistent leading spike when generalized spike-wave complexes are recorded. It is not unusual to see leading spikes alternate between the hemispheres. In these cases it may be impossible to determine which hemisphere contains the generator for the focal discharges. An activation procedure (sleep deprivation, sedated sleep) may settle the issue.

Sometimes, in those with intractable epilepsy, invasive recording is required to define the focus (preparatory for possible epilepsy surgery).

### Midline spikes

We often say that, during drowsiness or sleep, any sharp potential discharge occurring at one of the midline electrodes should be regarded as a normal phenomenon (vertex sharp waves) unless proven otherwise. The midline spike is a notable exception. This focal discharge with maximum focality at Fz, Cz, or Pz is thought to originate from the mesial surface of one of the cerebral hemispheres. It is difficult to determine whether the spike is right- or left-sided. Lateral spread of the potential field to C3 or C4 may give a clue. Note, however, that vertex sharp waves may be asymmetric as well, or show alternating lateralization. Of importance is that the technician accurately measures electrode placement. If midline spikes occur during wakefulness or light drowsiness, there should be no problem.

A practical observation: try comparing a suspicious discharge with undoubted symmetrical vertex activity. The latter usually have stereotyped waveforms, whereas the spike discharges will have a different morphology. Thus, identification of the "odd man out" is usually possible.

### Hypsarrhythmia

This distinctive EEG pattern is found in infants with West syndrome (infantile spasms). The term means "mountainous arrhythmia" and is characterized by a continual, generalized, very high voltage, chaotic pattern of slow waves, spikes and sharp waves. The spikes and sharp waves are multifocal, varying from moment to moment. Occasionally, generalized spikes are recorded. Spasms (Salaam attacks) may occur during the EEG. If so, there usually is a brief cessation of the hypsarrhythmic pattern with depression of the background with appearance of beta activity (electrodecremental response). On the other hand there may be no EEG change. In many cases hypsarrhythmia is self-limited. Treatment with steroids may suppress the pattern and terminate the seizures. There is little effect, however, on the patient's cognitive function. Among the newer antiepileptic drugs, vigabatrine has shown promise.

# 4

# THE EEG AND EPILEPSY

## EIGHT IMPORTANT EPILEPSY SYNDROMES

Following are brief discussions of eight important epilepsy syndromes along with the principal electrographic findings. Syndromic diagnosis confers a considerable advantage to the clinician in that it relates the clinical history and examination to EEG and imaging findings, prognosis, heritable characteristics and, in many cases, appropriate treatment.

### Simple Febrile Convulsions

Simple febrile convulsions generally occur between ages 6 months and 3 years. The events may be generalized tonic-clonic, tonic, or clonic in character. Duration is usually brief and should not be more than 15 minutes. The neurological examination is normal. The EEG usually contains no epileptiform activity, although spike-wave discharges and photosensitivity have been reported in some cases. Occipital delta waves have been reported in about one-third, and 1 percent eventually develop epilepsy – comparable to the general population.

### Complex Febrile Convulsions

These seizures are longer in duration than the above, that is, greater than 15 minutes. There usually are focal manifestations, and recurrence within 24 hours is common. The neurological examination is abnormal, and there often is a history of seizures in parents and siblings. The risk of subsequent epilepsy is higher than in simple febrile convulsions. Unfortunately, there is no reliable EEG correlate: the record may be normal or contain epileptiform activity of various types.

### West Syndrome (Infantile Spasms)

This serious illness of infancy typically has its onset at 3 to 7 months, and nearly always before the age of 2 years. The typical seizures consist of sudden, brief flexion movements of the body with flexion of the neck and abduction of the arms (so-called Salaam seizures). Extension of the neck and lower extremities may occur. The attacks are frequent and are associated with regression of milestones. Causes include cerebral malformations (agyria, pachygyria), perinatal brain damage, tuberous sclerosis, and a variety of metabolic disorders (e.g. aminoacidurias).

The typical EEG feature is hypsarrhythmia, a more or less continuous, high-voltage, chaotic, slow wave pattern with included multifocal spikes and sharp waves (see above). Over time there often is a change in the discharges, which may become focal. About half of the patients develop Lennox–Gastaut syndrome, and 80 percent mental retardation. Treatment is difficult. Valproate and vigabatrine may be tried, and some may respond to a benzodiazepine. Steroids have been used but are often poorly tolerated.

## Lennox–Gastaut Syndrome (LGS)

The Lennox–Gastaut Syndrome (LGS) has its onset in early childhood, usually around ages 3 to 5 years. Cardinal symptoms are mental retardation and multiple seizure types. The latter include tonic, atonic, and myoclonic events as well as so-called atypical absence attacks. The latter are of much longer duration than typical absence seizures, and indeed non-convulsive status epilepticus may occur, taking up many hours in the day.

A family history of epilepsy may be found. About one-third are of unknown cause, the remainder being due to congenital malformations, tuberous sclerosis, encephalitis, and perinatal hypoxic brain damage.

The EEG typically demonstrates a pattern of generalized slow spike-wave discharges at an average of 2 Hz (A-49). In addition, multifocal discharges are not uncommon. During slow wave sleep repeated electrographic seizures may occur consisting of a generalized rapid frequency at about 10 Hz.

Treatment of the seizures is difficult. Adrenocorticotropic hormone (ACTH), the ketogenic diet, and benzodiazepines (e.g. clobazam – unavailable in the US but available elsewhere, e.g. Canada) have all been used with variable success. Vigabatrine, one of the newer anti-epileptic drugs (AEDs), has shown promise, as has felbamate. The latter drug is recommended only when other modalities fail due to its bone marrow and hepatic toxicity.

Prognosis is generally poor, and the majority suffer from severe mental retardation, even if the seizures are eventually controlled.

## Absence Epilepsy

Absence epilepsy usually makes its appearance at the time the child enters school at about age 5 years, with a range between 4 and 8 years. These children are normal in every way, without evidence of cognitive or neurological deficits. The attacks themselves consist of staring episodes, with or without eye blinking, and generally are not longer than 10 seconds in duration. Minor automatisms appear in about 30 percent of cases, and occasional clonic or tonic features may be observed. Hyperventilation increases the likelihood of seizure occurrence, and pediatric neurologists routinely carry out the procedure in their offices in suspected cases. In the untreated state, hundreds of seizures may occur in a single day. There often is a family history of absence attacks, and twin studies have demonstrated a 75 to 80 percent concordance for the seizures and the EEG trait.

The EEG is characteristic, demonstrating generalized 3 (± 0.5) Hz spike-wave discharges that occur in highly rhythmic runs with a bifrontal preponderance (A-42). The background rhythms are entirely normal. During the events the child is unresponsive but recovers immediately upon discharge cessation. At the same time the normal background rhythms are restored without evidence of post-ictal slowing. During sleep there is distortion of the generalized discharges – the frequency band declines, and polyspike-wave complexes are not uncommon.

Treatment is gratifying for the clinician. A number of AEDs including ethosuximide, valproate, lamotrigine, and topiramate are likely to lead to complete seizure suppression. Compounds effective mainly in localization-related epilepsy such as phenytoin and carbamazepine should not be used in this condition. A note: if generalized tonic-clonic seizures coexist with absence attacks, ethosuximide monotherapy should not be used. Choose one of the other compounds mentioned above.

## Benign Childhood Epilepsy with Centro-temporal Spikes (BECTS)

This common epilepsy syndrome is easily recognized and, because of its favorable outlook, pediatric neurologists are pleased when they encounter a case. Onset is usually in late childhood or early adolescence. Imaging studies are normal; in fact, some authorities suggest that ordering such studies is not required when the diagnosis is clear. The neurological examination is normal, as is the EEG background. There may be a family history, and some have suggested an autosomal dominant gene.

The clinical seizures are characteristic. Common features include vocalization with guttural sounds, hypersalivation, oral sensations, and clenching of the teeth. There may be hemifacial movements, hemiconvulsions, and even generalized tonic-clonic convulsions.

Epileptiform discharges consist of sharp waves, often biphasic in configuration, occurring independently in the centro-temporal regions (C3/4–T3/4) (A-48). The discharges may occur in wakefulness, but are usually markedly activated by drowsiness and sleep. Isolated sharp waves while awake often transform into grouped or rhythmic discharges during sleep, and often alternate between the two hemispheres. There may be a left or right preponderance. Strictly unilateral discharges may also be seen. Rarely, some patients will have brief generalized discharges as well. Note that the EEG may contain many discharges although few seizures have ever occurred.

The prognosis is excellent. The seizures usually subside by mid-adolescence, and are uncommon after age 20 years. There is no universal agreement on treatment. Considering the benign nature of the condition, the debate is whether to treat or not. If treatment is elected, a compound appropriate for localization-related epilepsy is recommended.

### Juvenile Myoclonic Epilepsy (JME)

Most epilepsy specialists are gratified when they make a diagnosis of juvenile myoclonic epilepsy (JME). This syndrome has characteristic historical and EEG findings as well as an excellent prognosis. Onset typically is in adolescence. Patients with JME are neurologically normal without evidence of abnormality on imaging studies. Seizure phenomena include generalized tonic-clonic convulsions and, importantly, myoclonic jerks upon arising or soon thereafter. Multiple myoclonic jerks may lead to a generalized seizure. There is a genetic predisposition, and a putative gene has been proposed. The EEG demonstrates rapid, irregular, generalized spike-wave discharges. The seizures are usually well controlled with valproate, and there is evidence that two of the newer AEDs, lamotrigine and topiramate, are also effective.

A particular feature of the syndrome should be emphasized: treatment must be continued indefinitely, as relapse after discontinuation of AEDs is essentially inevitable.

### Benign Epilepsy of Childhood with Occipital Paroxysms

This syndrome is another example of a benign partial epilepsy – a diagnosis that is relatively easy and gratifying to make. Onset is usually at age 5 to 7 years, although seizures it may present in early childhood or adolescence. The seizures are characterized by visual symptoms such as flashing lights or even formed hallucinations. Following are automatisms as the seizure discharge spreads anteriorly to involve temporal structures. Headache is sometimes a feature of the paroxysmal event. These children are neurologically normal, and imaging studies are unrevealing. The EEG demonstrates high-voltage occipital spikes during the resting state with eyes closed. The discharges occur either in isolation or in rhythmic runs. With eye opening the discharges are attenuated but soon reappear after eye closure. The syndrome carries a good prognosis for complete seizure control.

## THE VALUE OF THE EEG IN EPILEPSY PROGNOSIS

Many clinicians place great value on the EEG when deciding whether or not to discontinue antiepileptic medication in seizure-free patients. This is a relatively complicated topic and will be reviewed only briefly. Although it seems obvious that an epileptiform EEG should stay one's hand from discontinuing AEDs, the correlation of potential seizure recurrence and the presence of discharges is not consistent. Many studies have been published, with varying results. A benchmark for considering discontinuation is 3 years of seizure freedom, although this varies from 2 to 5 years depending on the particular study.

Some have pointed to the weak correlation between probability of recurrence and the EEG findings. A reasonable summary would be that many factors appear to determine prognosis after discontinuation of AEDs including duration of seizure freedom, presence or absence of a structural lesion, duration of epilepsy, neurological findings, and age.

In adults, a good rule of thumb is that the patient, after 3 years of seizure freedom, has a 40 to 50 percent chance of remaining seizure-free after slow withdrawal of medication (a notable exception is juvenile myoclonic epilepsy (q.v.)). If the patient with partial onset epilepsy has an active spike focus, say in a temporal region, it appears that the chance of successful withdrawal is less. The lack of epileptiform activity on the EEG may point to a better chance of success, but this by no means is invariable. It would seem reasonable to continue AEDs in patients with active focal discharges. If patients with primary generalized epilepsy continue to display generalized spike-wave discharges, the probability of seizure recurrence is relatively high. In these cases medication should be continued. Note that even brief discharges of 1 to 2 seconds' duration are likely to correlate with very brief clinical lapses of which the patient is unaware. This has been confirmed by EEG monitoring studies of such patients when reaction times were determined during runs of generalized spike-wave discharges.

Other considerations are important, for example the patient's temperament and his or her occupation (is driving required?). The issue must be discussed in detail with the patient, offering the pros and cons of discontinuation. Some patients do not wish to take AEDs if not absolutely necessary and are willing to chance the possibility of seizure recurrence. They may say that a recurrence will satisfy them of the necessity for resuming AEDs. Others are quite fearful of a possible seizure and are adamant about remaining on AEDs. As with all physician–patient interactions, a mutual understanding is essential for arriving at an individualized plan that is acceptable to both parties. The situation appears to be different in children; there is evidence that continuing EEG epileptiform activity, among other factors, is a predictor of seizure recurrence after stopping AEDs. This applies both to focal and generalized discharges.

## EPILEPSY MONITORING

EEG-video monitoring is the "gold standard" of epilepsy diagnosis. Whereas, in most cases, the diagnosis of epilepsy rests on the clinical history, there are many exceptions. These arise due to incomplete historical data, for example lack of a clear description of the events in question, or a patient who reports unobserved blackouts or loss of consciousness. Monitoring is most often used to establish the diagnosis, but there are other purposes:

- characterization of attacks in a person with known epilepsy;
- determination of seizure frequency in those with frequent complex partial or absence seizures;

- determination of the frequency of epileptiform discharges;
- distinguishing between epileptic and non-epileptic seizures;
- guidance of treatment; and
- investigation of reflex epilepsies.

If the reported spontaneous events have a frequency of weekly or less often, prolonged EEG-video monitoring in an inpatient unit may be productive. Patients may stay in the monitoring unit for days, or up to a week or more, in anticipation of recording a paroxysmal event on EEG and videotape. If events are more frequent, say daily or three times weekly, out-patient monitoring may be sufficient to establish a diagnosis or characterize the events. This procedure typically continues for 6 to 8 hours and is cost-effective. Various provocation techniques are carried out during the study, including hyperventilation, photic stimulation, provocation (see section on non-epileptic seizures), and sleep. Note that sleep deprivation before the study is useful and serves to increase the probability of seizure occurrence. The hit rate under these circumstances is on the order of 60 percent.

**Ambulatory EEG (AEEG) Monitoring**

This long-term monitoring technique has the attraction of sending the patient home with a small, portable EEG amplifier and recorder. Typically, the patient carries out normal activities and keeps a diary of his or her activities and any events that occur. Recording may be carried out for days, or a week or more. The patient returns to the EEG department daily for a change of cassette. A drawback of AEEG is the excessive artifact that mars recording when a motor event occurs.

This makes difficult (if not impossible) the differentiation of epileptic from psychogenic non-epileptic seizures on the basis of the recorded event. In these circumstances the observations of others – parents, partners, and even workmates – may be helpful. If interictal spikes are recorded, however, the possibility of the seizure being epileptic becomes more likely. By contrast, absence attacks are usually quite evident on AEEG and may be counted with some accuracy. Another useful aspect of the procedure is recording during a night's sleep. During drowsiness and sleep, artifact is much reduced, and focal spikes or generalized discharges may become evident. Such findings would support a diagnosis of epilepsy in patients with spells of uncertain nature.

# THE EEG IN NON-EPILEPTIC SEIZURES OF PSYCHOGENIC ORIGIN

The EEG is an indispensable tool in the diagnosis of non-epileptic seizures (NES) of psychogenic origin. Included are routine EEGs during which a NES occurs spontaneously or is precipitated through techniques of suggestion, and EEG-video monitoring studies. An important observation: the routine EEG in subjects with NES may be normal or abnormal. In fact, about 20 percent of patients with NES also suffer from epileptic seizures. In these cases, epileptiform discharges are not uncommon. Thus, the presence of interictal spikes in the EEG does not differentiate the two. When NES are recorded (especially the generalized motor variety that mimick generalized tonic convulsions) the EEG is dominated by high-voltage muscle and movement artifact. There are no premonitory spikes, nor is there evidence of a recruiting rhythm. During the motor activity, which often is discontinuous, one may see brief runs of alpha rhythm during brief quiet intervals, incompatible with a depressed state of consciousness. When the clinical seizure subsides there is no post-ictal slowing and alpha is re-established – this despite the fact that the patient may still be unresponsive. Staring spells or minor motor activities resembling complex partial seizures sometimes characterize NES. In these circumstances the EEG contains no lateralized or generalized slowing, or epileptiform activity. Indeed, alpha is usually noted during the spell.

Exceptions to the rule that the lack of EEG epileptiform activity supports a diagnosis of NES are the simple partial seizure (SPS) and a seizure originating from the mesial frontal cortex. In only about one-fourth of true SPS cases is associated focal ictal activity recorded with scalp electrodes. Thus, the lack of ictal activity during suspected focal motor or sensory NES would not lend support to the diagnosis. With respect to seizures of mesial frontal origin, a recruiting response may not spread to the convexity and thus elude recording by scalp electrodes. In some cases, recording with a transverse bipolar montage may reveal a midline spike at Fz or Cz. When EEG findings are lacking, the diagnosis must rest on clinical grounds, for example duration, physiological progression, and stereotypy.

## STATUS EPILEPTICUS

### Generalized Convulsive Status Epilepticus (GCSE)

Generalized convulsive status epilepticus (GCSE, formerly Grand Mal Status) can be divided into two distinct types: overt and subtle. This is a useful categorization in that the two are closely related but have quite different clinical manifestations, EEG findings, and prognosis.

### *Overt GCSE*

This is the easiest to identify and is familiar to most. There are various definitions. For example, in the epidemiological literature, convulsive activity for at least 30 minutes defines GCSE. As a practical matter we adhere to the following definition, which is useful in clinical practice:

1. Two or more generalized tonic-clonic convulsions (GTCC) without complete recovery of cognitive function between events (there may be unilateral post-ictal paresis if the seizure is secondarily generalized, which in adults is

usually the case). If there is complete recovery of cognitive function before the next seizure occurs, we refer to this state as serial seizures.

2. Sustained convulsive activity lasting 10 minutes (the usual GTC has a duration of about 1 minute).

(**Note**: if a prolonged convulsive seizure comes to your attention before 10 minutes have elapsed do not wait – start treatment at once.)

The authors concede that a GTC may be followed by a prolonged post-ictal state (confusion, memory deficits), say for an hour, followed by a second seizure. Should such a patient be said to be in status? One might well argue that this is not status in the usual sense. The temporal dividing line of status versus serial seizures with interval cognitive impairment is difficult to identify. Treatment of such patients should rely on clinical judgment, with intravenous treatment being suggested in most cases.

### Subtle GCSE

This is characterized by a comatose state with minor motor manifestations (e.g. multifocal myoclonic jerks, minor facial twitching, or nystagmoid jerking of the eyes), secondary to a catastrophic cerebral event such as anoxia. Alternatively, subtle status may evolve from prolonged overt status. The EEG demonstrates continual or discontinuous epileptiform activity, even periodic epileptiform discharges (PEDs, see below).

### EEG Findings in GCSE

Treiman and colleagues, supported by animal studies, have proposed five successive EEG changes during prolonged GCSE. It is stipulated that not all experts accept such an orderly progression of EEG findings in generalized convulsive status (see References). Nonetheless, what follows is a useful way to look at the problem.

The first stage is repeated, discrete clinico-electrographic seizures with typical EEG manifestations including a rapid recruiting rhythm, starting with generalized or focal discharges, followed by a generalized interference pattern and synchronous high-voltage spike-wave discharges at an average frequency of 2.5 to 3 Hz (Figure 4-1). Before the patient recovers full cognitive function the second seizure occurs.

The second stage is the merging pattern – that is, polymorphic electrographic seizure activity – spike-waves interrupted by rhythmic waves of various frequencies that wax and wane in amplitude (Figure 4-2). The patient continues in the comatose state and is usually not clinically convulsing. This state may emerge within a relatively short time. After initial treatment, and without the benefit of EEG recording, the patient may be deemed "cured" of status because convulsive movements have ceased. Nothing could be farther from the truth. Minor motor

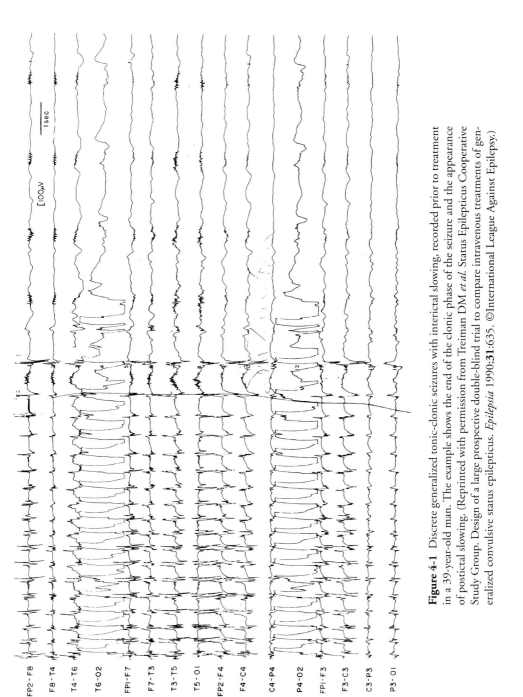

**Figure 4-1** Discrete generalized tonic-clonic seizures with interictal slowing, recorded prior to treatment in a 39-year-old man. The example shows the end of the clonic phase of the seizure and the appearance of postictal slowing. (Reprinted with permission from Treiman DM *et al.* Status Epilepticus Cooperative Study Group. Design of a large prospective double-blind trial to compare intravenous treatments of generalized convulsive status epilepticus. *Epilepsia* 1990;**31**:635. ©International League Against Epilepsy.)

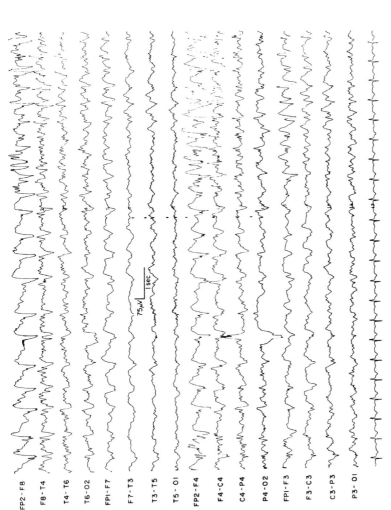

**Figure 4-2** Merging of discrete seizures, recorded prior to treatment in a 64-year-old man. Ictal discharges are continuous, but with waxing and waning of frequency and amplitude. An increase in frequency and amplitude can be seen beginning on the right side of the recording. (Reprinted with permission from Treiman DM, *et al.* Status Epilepticus Cooperative Study Group. Design of a large prospective double-blind trial to compare intravenous treatments of generalized convulsive status epilepticus. *Epilepsia* 1990;**31**:635. ©International League Against Epilepsy.)

manifestations such as myoclonic jerks or intermittent nystagmus may be observed but are not considered by many clinicians to represent continuing status. The reader will appreciate that status is defined by electrographic findings, not obvious convulsions.

The third stage is continuous electrographic ictal activity (Figure 4-3). Here, we have continuous generalized spike-wave discharges. Again, the patient is not clinically convulsing although minor motor manifestations may persist. The continuous electrographic seizure activity reveals why the patient does not awaken.

Following is the fourth stage of electrographic discharges interrupted by depressions of cerebral activity (so-called flat periods) (Figure 4-4). The suppressions herald the severe consequences of prolonged status. This picture suggests a poor prognosis.

In the fifth stage, high-voltage generalized periodic epileptiform discharges (PEDs) dominate the record. The discharges, synchronous slow or sharp potentials, occur every few seconds, and the patient is in serious trouble (Figure 4-5). Status has persisted much too long. Treatment needs to be commenced immediately if it is not already underway.

Outcome depends primarily on the underlying disease process. If the cause is cerebral anoxia, such patients rarely recover despite vigorous treatment. Outcome is usually death or, in some cases, marked neurological impairment, for example persistent vegetative state. If subtle status results from a prolonged period of overt GCSE, there is a better chance for survival. In any case, the patient always deserves prompt and aggressive treatment.

### Non-convulsive Status Epilepticus (NCSE)

Non-convulsive status epilepticus (NCSE) is a term of non-uniform definition. The literature of NCSE is confusing owing to the lack of agreed-upon terminology. Various terms referring to NCSE are found in the literature, for example twilight state and epileptic confusional state.

NCSE implies a seizure state characterized by altered consciousness, sometimes with minor motor manifestations. In some series of NCSE, cases of generalized convulsive status of the subtle type are mixed with cases of altered awareness that are not secondary to a catastrophic cerebral insult. The prognosis of these two states is quite different. The reader is advised to pay attention to the patient cohort in any article on this topic. For this discussion, NCSE is divided into two types: absence NCSE and complex partial NCSE.

#### *Absence NCSE*

In absence NCSE, most often encountered in children, the EEG is characterized by generalized, rhythmic spike-wave runs, most often encountered in children. The discharges, generalized at onset, are manifestations of primary

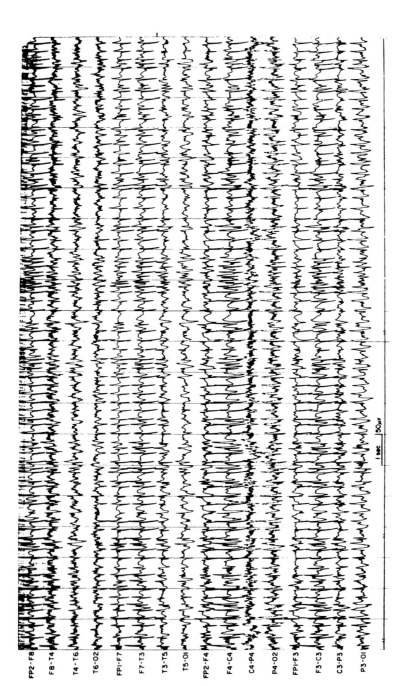

**Figure 4-3** Continuous ictal discharges recorded prior to treatment in a 53-year-old man. Continuous ictal activity persisted for more than 3.5 hours despite vigorous treatment with diazepam, lorazepam, phenytoin, and phenobarbital. (Reprinted with permission from Treiman DM. The role of benzodiazepines in the management of status epilepticus. *Neurology* 1990;**40**:990–994. © International League Against Epilepsy.)

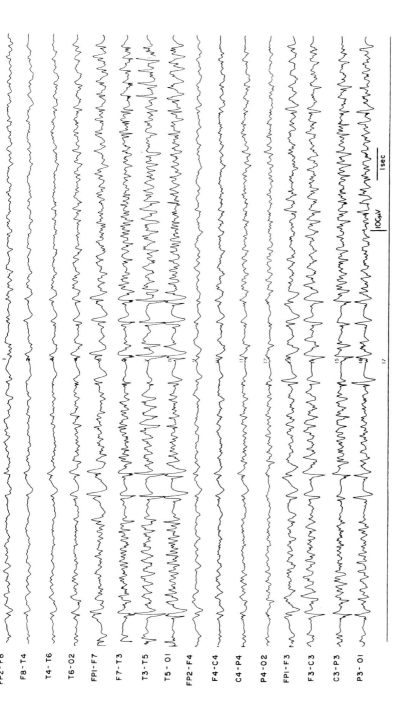

**Figure 4-4** Continuous ictal discharges with flat periods recorded prior to treatment in a 68-year-old man. The seizure focus is clearly in the left hemisphere, but the spread of ictal activity to the right hemisphere can be seen as well. (Reprinted with permission from Treiman DM *et al.* Status Epilepticus Cooperative Study Group. Design of a large prospective double-blind trial to compare intravenous treatments of generalized convulsive status epilepticus. *Epilepsia* 1990;**31**:635. © International League Against Epilepsy.)

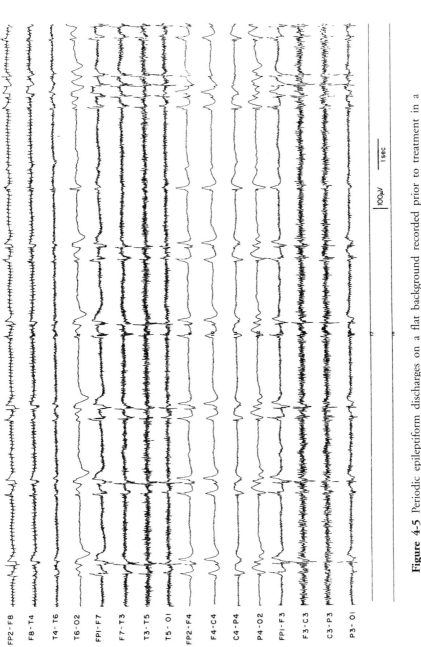

**Figure 4-5** Periodic epileptiform discharges on a flat background recorded prior to treatment in a 64-year-old man. (Reprinted with permission from Treiman DM, *et al.* Status Epilepticus Cooperative Study Group. Design of a large prospective double-blind trial to compare intravenous treatments of generalized convulsive status epilepticus. *Epilepsia* 1990;**31**:635. © International League Against Epilepsy.)

generalized epilepsy. The complexes are usually in the 3 Hz frequency band. The spike-wave runs (or trains) are usually discontinuous. When they subside, the background is relatively normal. The patient is clouded or unresponsive during the discharges. In some cases, absence status culminates in a generalized convulsion.

### Complex Partial NCSE

Complex Partial NCSE can be divided into two general types:

- those with repeated typical complex partial seizures without cognitive recovery between events; and
- those with persistent alteration of consciousness.

In the first type, the EEG demonstrates electrographic seizures originating in a temporal lobe, spreading to involve both hemispheres (A-46, A-47). Typically the seizure begins with a motionless stare followed by automatisms associated with altered awareness. Following the seizure the patient is confused. The second seizure occurs before recovery. If the complex partial seizure has a frontal origin, then vocalization and posturing may herald the event. At onset the EEG may reveal a new, rapid frequency in a frontal region. Automatisms may be absent or, on the other hand, consist of vigorous, generalized, and seemingly chaotic limb movements. Seizure frequency may be high, but there is usually cognitive recovery between events. Thus, the rubric of serial seizures would be more suitable than status. To the unwary such seizures appear to be non-epileptic in nature. EEG-video monitoring should settle the issue.

The second type is characterized by generalized epileptiform activity. Many varieties of waveform have been described, ranging from spikes and polyspikes to rhythmic frequencies, often sharply contoured in configuration. There is commonly a bifrontal amplitude preponderance, and the paroxysmal activity is usually discontinuous (A-50). When discharges temporarily subside the background is slow, but remnants of rhythmic activity are noted. The patient displays an altered mental status, ranging from some confusion, retaining responsiveness, to complete interruption of consciousness. In some cases the patient remains responsive, complaining only of some mental fuzziness or memory difficulty. The authors have observed a patient whose non-convulsive status was characterized only by a personality change (from outgoing to somewhat subdued) when the EEG showed repeated runs of ictal activity.

In many patients there may be little recovery during interictal periods, although waxing and waning of mental status is not unusual. Of importance is that a focal onset of the generalized discharges is seldom apparent. Only when status resolves may one discover a focal slow wave or sharp wave abnormality. Causes are diverse, but the condition often occurs in older patients after drug withdrawal (especially benzodiazepines and psychotropic agents) and during an intercurrent illness such as sepsis. If complex partial NCSE occurs in ill, hospitalized patients, the outcome may be poor, owing primarily to the underlying medical or neuro-logical illness. Note also that complex partial status is sometimes a cause of failure to regain consciousness after surgery. In such cases an EEG should be ordered if the patient does not recover as expected.

The alert reader will recognize that there may be an overlap between NCSE and subtle GCSE. If severe brain damage underlies the seizure activity, a diag-nosis of subtle GCSE would be appropriate. Some patients – particularly the elderly with severe associated medical illness – develop prolonged NCSE that is refractory to treatment. In such cases an ultimate transition from NCSE to subtle GCSE probably occurs, owing to underlying or developing brain damage.

# 5

# THE EEG IN OTHER NEUROLOGICAL AND MEDICAL CONDITIONS

## THE DEMENTIAS

### Alzheimer's Disease

In its early stages, Alzheimer's disease may display little or no EEG abnormality. As the disease progresses there first is slowing of the posterior rhythm with a gradual increase in diffuse slowing, initially in the theta range followed by increasing amounts of delta. Eventually the posterior rhythmic activity is lost (A-62). Focal findings may be evident if the process proceeds asymmetrically. Epileptiform discharges may appear later in the process. Note that clinical seizures, generalized or focal, become more common as the disease progresses – particularly in its late stages.

### Multi-infarct Dementia

Multi-infarct dementia (MID) is difficult to differentiate from Alzheimer's disease on clinical grounds, and also on EEG grounds. Some clues are available, however. In MID the record is more likely to display asymmetrical features, even focality. This no doubt results from multiple small strokes in the course of the illness. Rarely, pseudoperiodic discharges may appear, especially if the disease is severe, suggesting the possibility of Creutzfeldt–Jakob disease (CJD, see below). Usually, the differentiation can be made on clinical grounds as well as the lack of progression characteristic of CJD.

### Creutzfeldt–Jakob Disease (CJD)

Creutzfeldt–Jakob disease has distinctive EEG and clinical characteristics. In the first place, the disease is rapidly progressive with cognitive decline and parallel EEG changes. The background rhythms become fragmented and are destroyed. Diffuse slowing appears and increases. Later, the distinctive periodic sharp wave discharge is recorded (see section on periodicity and A-63). At first, the discharge may be more irregular and even focal, only later becoming generalized and synchronous. Background activity declines in amplitude. Eventually the EEG is dominated by the periodic discharges with no discernible background. Before death there is a decline in, and ultimate disappearance of, the discharges, leaving an essentially featureless record.

Heidenhain's variant of CJD is encountered infrequently. In this condition, the process begins in the posterior portions of the hemispheres, spreading to involve the brain as a whole. Periodic discharges likewise may appear first in the occipital regions. A clinical note: the appearance of periodicity is associated with clinical myoclonus. The latter may be subtle at first and missed by the clinician. Close examination of the patient will reveal the motor activity.

## Pick's Disease

Pick's disease deserves brief mention. This uncommon form of dementia with heritable characteristics, involves mainly the frontal and temporal lobes early in its course. Pick's disease is now classified as one of several fronto-temporal dementias. The EEG may reveal focal slowing in these areas. It is emphasized, however, that relatively little EEG experience is available in this condition.

# STROKE

It may come as a surprise to learn that the EEG contributes to the evaluation of patients with stroke, both ischemic and hemorrhagic. Although imaging studies (MRI/CT) remain the key diagnostic investigations, the combination of anatomical and physiological data increases our understanding of the pathological process in question.

## Ischemic Stroke

Many patients presenting with acute ischemic stroke are relatively easy to diagnose on clinical grounds with respect to the event itself as well as its location. (Note to our readers: the neurological examination still retains its importance!) Others are less straightforward, and the clinician depends on an imaging study to aid in accurate diagnosis. In the acute phase (say, the first 24 hours) the CT scan may be of little help, and an MRI may not be readily available. In such cases the EEG offers data of interest. For example, the usual EEG picture in cases of middle cerebral artery occlusion reveals an irregular or polymorphic delta focus in the involved hemisphere, maximal in frontal, temporal and parietal regions. Rhythmic delta runs may be admixed. In addition, the posterior dominant rhythm is usually disrupted.

When edema supervenes the slowing may be more profound. Indeed, if the patient is lethargic, possibly due to midline intracranial shift, the opposite hemisphere will also demonstrate slowing and disorganization. Associated increased ICP may be accompanied by bifrontal intermittent rhythmic delta waves (FIRDA).

With resolution of acute changes, there is gradual decline in the slow wave focus, which becomes intermittent and may resolve completely. At this point the record will demonstrate depression of background activity in the involved regions. Look especially for depression of beta activity, perhaps associated with a modest degree of slowing. During sleep, unilateral depression of sleep spindles and vertex sharp waves may provide additional evidence of the infarct.

Branch occlusions of the middle cerebral artery present a more limited EEG abnormality, as might be expected. If the parietal branch is involved, findings may be few – perhaps consisting of preponderant theta activity over the involved area (A-60).

Occipital strokes present a different picture. Slowing over the posterior temporal and occipital regions may be evident along with destruction of the alpha. As with any acute infarct, the presence of edema may provoke a more widespread abnormality. Chronically, the record may simply show absence or near absence of the alpha. Note that photic stimulation may evoke an asymmetric following response with depression over the involved side.

Occlusion of the anterior cerebral artery usually results in frontal slowing, with or without projected rhythmic delta on the involved side. Alternatively, the projected delta may appear bifrontally with lateralization to the side of the infarct. In such cases the occipital rhythms are preserved.

In some patients with acute infarction a few sharp potentials may be recorded. Further, the EEG sometimes reveals a pattern of periodic lateralized epileptiform discharges (PLEDs, see section on periodicity).

Many strokes are subcortical with sparing of the overlying cortex. Lacunar strokes involving the internal capsule or basal ganglia are common in patients with hypertension and are not always easy to differentiate clinically from those with cortical/subcortical involvement. Instead of demonstrating focal slowing, the record in these patients is usually normal. Alternatively, it may contain a mild diffuse abnormality without lateralizing features. In either case, the likelihood of a subcortical process is great.

A final note. Patients with clinically diagnosed transient ischemic attacks are often referred for an EEG. In these cases the record is usually normal or non-focal if obtained after resolution of the neurological findings. In some cases, however, intermittent focal slowing may be evident, suggesting that residual cerebral dysfunction is indeed present despite a normal neurological examination. If the EEG is obtained while the patient is symptomatic, appropriate focal or lateralized slowing will be evident.

## Hemorrhagic Stroke

Hemorrhagic strokes present a highly variable EEG picture depending on the site of involvement, extent of the pathology, and the patient's state of awareness.

A relatively small hemorrhage in the centrum semiovale likely results in a minor degree of lateralized slowing – or even no clear lateralization. On the other hand, deep ganglionic hemorrhages, usually associated with obtundation, demonstrate marked disruption of electrocortical activity with bilateral delta activity. Lateralization to the involved side may be seen, although in the face of depressed consciousness any asymmetry may not be evident. Bifrontal delta activity is common in such cases.

## SUBDURAL HEMATOMA

Before the advent of imaging, the EEG was the most important first-line study for the diagnosis of subdural hematoma (SDH). EEG findings suggestive of SDH aided the clinician in planning definitive studies such as arteriography. Today, the mainstay of diagnosing SDH is the CT scan, but in some instances the EEG can play an important role. Take, for example, an elderly person with no history of head trauma who becomes somewhat more confused than usual. There are a number of diagnostic possibilities, including metabolic derangement, an unobserved seizure, progressive dementia and, indeed, a subdural hematoma.

The classic EEG finding in SDH is depression of cerebral activity over the involved hemisphere. This so-called insulation defect consists of reduced amplitude of the background as compared to the opposite hemisphere. This often is particularly evident with respect to beta activity. In addition, the posterior dominant rhythm or alpha may be disrupted or even absent (A-61). If the collection is large associated slowing may be evident. It should be emphasized that there is considerable variability in the EEG picture, and the classic finding of background depression is not always seen. If the SDH is small there may be no obvious EEG findings. On the other hand, the record is usually abnormal with larger collections, even though the classic findings may not be present.

We also find unilateral depression of cerebral activity in subdural hygroma and atrophic processes secondary to congenital brain damage. In addition, porencephalopathy leads to striking depression of the background that may present an essentially isopotential (flat) picture.

## METABOLIC DISORDERS

The EEG can make a contribution to the diagnosis of metabolic encephalopathies. Importantly, the patient's progress can be followed with serial EEGs. This is of interest in that resolution of electrographic changes lags behind correction of the underlying metabolic abnormality. Residual findings in such cases help to explain why the patient has not fully recovered, even though his or her biochemical parameters have returned to normal.

### General EEG Features

The hallmark of a metabolic encephalopathy is diffuse slowing. In addition, the posterior dominant rhythm (PDR) is invariably disrupted and slowed, or is essentially absent. The slowing may be mild or profound, depending on the extent of the encephalopathy and the level of consciousness. It usually is symmetrical unless there is an underlying focal cerebral lesion unrelated to the metabolic disorder. In such cases one may see focal as well as diffuse slowing. During recording, the technologist should attempt to arouse the patient. This may result in an increase in the background frequency – a demonstration of EEG reactivity – offering some support for metabolic derangement.

In addition to diffuse slowing, FIRDA may be recorded, implying involvement of the deep midline structures by the metabolic process. Note that FIRDA is also seen in intoxications, increased ICP and deep frontal lesions. It is therefore non-specific (A-56).

To summarize, the usual progression of EEG changes in metabolic disorders are as follows:

1. In early stages there is slowing of the posterior dominant rhythm with scattered theta frequencies.
2. Later, there is increased slowing in theta and delta ranges with disruption of the posterior dominant rhythm.
3. Frontal intermittent rhythmic delta activity (FIRDA) may then appear.
4. Triphasic waves are a later development (see below).
5. Finally, there is marked generalized slowing with depression of amplitude.

### The Triphasic Wave in Hepatic and Renal Encephalopathies

An important feature of metabolic encephalopathies is the triphasic wave. The three phases of this waveform sometimes are not evident, and biphasic waves are commonly seen as well. Triphasic activity is synchronous and most prominent in the frontal derivations (A-58). At its fullest development, triphasic activity is nearly continuous and highly rhythmic. A classic etiology is hepatic encephalopathy. It is said that true triphasic waves, recorded with a wide potential field, demonstrate an A-P delay; that is, the frontal component leads the posterior component by 100 ms or so, though in the authors' experience this phenomenon is not always apparent. The underlying neurophysiological reason for front to back delay is not well understood.

The alert reader will observe that the triphasic wave bears a close resemblance to the epileptiform sharp wave. In fact, it sometimes is difficult to differentiate a metabolic encephalopathy with prominent triphasic activity from non-convulsive status epilepticus (NCSE). The two conditions may have strikingly similar EEG appearances (there is no A-P delay with the discharges of NCSE). A good clue in deciding which condition obtains is the frequently occurring discontinuity in the runs of discharges in NCSE. When ongoing epileptiform discharges subside, even for a brief period, a relatively low-voltage background is revealed, sometimes with rhythmic or quasi-rhythmic waves. This finding provides support for NCSE and militates against a metabolic etiology.

Triphasic waves are not pathognomonic of hepatic encephalopathy. These potentials also occur in other metabolic problems, for example renal failure. Overall, the triphasic activity is not as well developed or persistent in non-hepatic processes as it is in hepatic encephalopathy. Note that hepatic encephalopathy accounts for more than half the recordings with triphasic waves, followed by renal failure in about one third. In both renal and hepatic encephalopathies spike and sharp wave discharges, perhaps multifocal, are sometimes recorded. Note that seizures may occur in both conditions.

### Other Metabolic Encephalopathies

With metabolic encephalopathies, triphasic and biphasic waves may be seen, but other phenomena are more common. For example, in hypocalcemia, both diffuse slowing and epileptiform discharges are characteristic. When calcium concentrations reach the neighborhood of 5 mg/dL or less, multifocal and even synchronous spikes may result. Background activity is typically disrupted. The spikes resolve with correction of the metabolic defect. In hypercalcemia the cardinal finding is marked slowing with high-amplitude, sharply contoured bifrontal delta waves.

Spikes are associated with hypomagnesemia, although low magnesium levels are often associated with hypocalcemia. Severe hyponatremia may result in seizures with concomitant multifocal spikes. Hypoglycemia similarly produces multifocal spikes, and focal onset electrographic seizures may be recorded. Triphasic waves are occasionally recorded. Correction of the metabolic defect results in normalization of the EEG. No imaging correlate of focal seizure activity is found.

Hypothyroidism, presenting as cognitive slowing, usually results in slowing of the PDR along with some degree of diffuse slowing. There usually are no associated epileptiform discharges.

## COMA

The EEG in coma varies markedly with the underlying cause. At one end of the spectrum is cerebral anoxia. In this case, the record may demonstrate isopotentiality, a burst-suppression pattern (with or without included spikes), or periodic epileptiform discharges (PEDs). Indeed, the picture may be that of GCSE of the subtle type (see section on status).

Alpha coma and theta coma are distinctive EEG findings, usually resulting from pervasive cerebral damage (as from anoxia with development of laminar necrosis involving layers 4 and 5). In these cases, the rhythmic alpha or theta frequencies characteristically appear most prominently in the frontal derivations, but may be diffusely represented. There is no response to external stimuli or passive opening of the eyes. These findings imply a very poor prognosis despite the apparent normal appearance of the record. This emphasizes the importance of knowing the patient's state of awareness in order properly to interpret the EEG.

Metabolic derangement also results in coma. Triphasic activity has been mentioned above, but in many cases (regardless of cause) the picture is one of amplitude depression with diffuse slowing. Non-convulsive status (NCSE) presents with a wide range of alteration of consciousness including coma. Although there frequently are clinical clues such as intermittent nystagmus or minor myoclonic activity, the patient may simply be unresponsive (see EEG findings in the section on NCSE).

/

# 6

# TIPS ON READING AND REPORTING THE EEG

The novice is confronted by a dizzying array of wiggly lines in a seemingly endless series of displays (or pages). At first the task seems impossible. How can I ever master this arcane science (or art, or a combination of both)? The secret, as in most complicated matters, is to break the EEG down to its essential elements. At the end of the exercise, one reassembles the parts to make a cohesive, understandable whole. We think of it as providing the ordering clinician with a well-wrapped package, bow and all. After all, the whole point of EEG interpretation is to help the clinician in his or her diagnostic quest.

## ELEMENTS OF THE REPORT

One method of designing the EEG report breaks it down into five sections. Each is important in constructing an accurate picture of the patient's electrophysiological status.

1. Clinical Information. This section should include the reason for the EEG request. The clinical information supplied by the clinician is often rudimentary; thus, the technician can be of assistance in obtaining additional information from the patient and/or the patient's chart. If the patient had a recent seizure, say hours or a day before recording, it should be indicated here. If the patient is taking medications that have effects on the brain, they should be listed here. Examples include AEDs, psychotropic agents, and sedatives.

2. Conditions of Recording. In this section, describe whether the EEG is obtained under special circumstances such as after sleep deprivation or sedation. Then indicate the technician's estimate of the patient's state – awake, drowsy, sleeping, lethargic, comatose, etc. Other observations by the technician should be noted: the patient might have been restless, tense, confused, moving throughout, chewing, etc. If the record was obtained at the

bedside, or in an ICU or emergency room, it should be indicated here. All these features set the stage for understanding the following section.

3. Factual Report. Here, cerebral and non-cerebral events are described. We like to think that this section creates a word picture that more or less accurately lays out the important findings. Bear in mind that the report may be read by another electroencephalographer, and the record itself may be reviewed. Ask yourself, would such a peer reviewer come to the same conclusion? Another way to look at the issue is to ask, could I show a slide of this apparent spike or sharp wave at a national meeting without fear of being hooted off the stage?

4. Impression. State in brief summary the essential findings. For example: "This is an abnormal EEG demonstrating, against a normal background, an active spike focus in the anterior temporal region." Or: "Abnormal EEG owing to mild, diffuse slowing along with intermittent right temporal delta activity."

5. Clinical Correlation. This final section is perhaps the most important aspect of the report. It is a truism that the average clinician does not read the detail in the factual report, nor does he or she much care whether there is mu rhythm over the left central region. The clinician wants diagnostic help, if possible. The authors look at it this way: the factual report is important for electroencephalographers; the impression and clinical correlation is of interest to clinicians. So, one offers as much assistance in this section as possible. If the findings support a diagnosis of localization related epilepsy, say it here. If the findings are consistent with a metabolic disorder, or an acute infarct, then so indicate. This section is also the place to recommend further studies, if indicated. For example, if there is a minor temporal abnormality in a patient with probable complex partial seizures, you may suggest an EEG after sleep deprivation. Or, you might recommend an ambulatory EEG. Remember, serial studies are often helpful in certain situations (metabolic disorders, for example). The clinician needs your guidance in ordering immediate additional testing and how he or she should proceed in the future.

A further consideration is what to do when the record is studded with artifacts. Adhering to the principle of aiding the clinician, one should try to make some helpful statement even though, as a whole, the record is unsatisfactory for accurate interpretation. A few pages of relatively quiescent recording may reveal focal slow waves, or even a spike or two, giving some clue concerning the clinical problem. In these cases, one may recommend a repeat tracing when the patient is less confused or less restless, or perhaps a tracing after mild sedation, before a final impression is rendered.

## HOW TO LOOK AT THE RECORD

In order to interpret the record properly, one must have clearly in mind the elements of a normal EEG. This establishes a template, against which all deviations are to be compared. In the case of adults, recall that the normal waking record contains an alpha rhythm (with some exceptions as outlined previously), of maximum amplitude in the posterior quadrants. Beta activity is present fronto-centrally, in greater or lesser amounts. A few theta frequencies are acceptable if not lateralized. Little else is present. The response to hyperventilation may be marked in younger adults. Consistent lateralization is not permitted. A following (driving) response to intermittent photic stimulation is variable, but there should be no activation of epileptiform activity. The elements of drowsiness and sleep round out the template of the normal adult record.

It is sometimes useful to analyze carefully the first few interpretable pages or 10-second digital epochs. (Bear in mind that it may take several minutes before the patient settles down and relaxes fully.) This exercise is often time well spent. One may appreciate a hint of focality, or a hint of paroxysmal activity, or a possible asymmetry of background activity. In any event such analysis can set the stage for more rapid analysis of subsequent recording, providing clues on what to look for. Another hint that often pays dividends is to divide reading into vertical and horizontal appraisals.

Horizontal reading appraises and compares channels on the left side of the head with those on the right by scanning the record from left to right, choosing, for example, the left and right temporal leads followed by the left and right paracentral leads.

Vertical reading, scanning a particular segment of a second or so from top to bottom, concentrates more on particular waveforms and their distributions. A common problem with the beginner is that he or she becomes enmeshed in the complicated polyrhythmicity of the EEG by reading only vertically. This results in confusion and overreading. Overreading is a pitfall to be avoided (as, to some extent, is underreading), but more on this later.

Reading horizontally reveals abnormalities that may not be at all evident when reading vertically. In essence, horizontal reading reveals the broad picture presented by the EEG. For example, this is the best way to determine alpha asymmetry. One can easily determine alpha asymmetries, abundance, and irregularities. This is not evident with vertical reading. Unilateral or bilateral slowing also becomes more evident during horizontal reading. Importantly, the appearance of a new, paroxysmal frequency, diagnostic of an electrographic seizure, may not be evident with vertical reading. Many cases of recurrent electrographic seizures have been missed due to this oversight.

Now, look for pages where the patient is in his or her most alert state. Here is the point to analyze the alpha rhythm or the PDR. Is it well organized (that is, nicely rhythmic, devoid of admixed slower frequencies), or is it irregular or poorly persistent, or variable in frequency? Analysis of the PDR helps materially to determine laterality of any unilateral pathology. It is emphasized that if the patient is not maximally alert, no definite determination can be made of a PDR asymmetry.

Now, evaluate the beta rhythm. Beta offers a few clues to the presence of pathology. If asymmetric, it usually points to pathology on the side of diminished amplitude. If abundant, it may reveal a drug effect. In any case, it is an important aspect of the basic or resting record.

The next task is to determine the presence of slow waves in the background. The slowing may be diffuse – that is, not lateralized and non-focal. Look for both theta and delta frequencies. Is there a small amount of intermittent theta activity? A great deal of theta? Are there mainly delta waves? A combination of the two? We sometimes look at the broad picture and try to decide if it belongs in the theta box or the delta box! Note that slowing may be more or less continuous, discontinuous, paroxysmal, rhythmic, or arrhythmic. There may be variable but inconsistent lateralization.

One problem is to determine at the outset whether or not there is excess slowing – that is, how much is too much? This is a somewhat subjective call. Major determinants include age and state, and the reader must constantly bear these factors in mind. Look for pages in which the patient is fully awake. (If the patient is drowsy throughout, this may not be possible.) Most electroencephalographers accept a small amount of theta in the background of adults as normal (say up to 5%) – mainly in the temporal regions.

Generally speaking, delta activity does not appear in the normal, waking adult EEG. Perhaps a few random low-voltage delta waves might be acceptable. Note that delta is common in the EEGs of children (see section on children). Also, in the elderly, delta waves are commonly recorded in the temporal derivations, indicative of some degree of cerebral pathology but not necessarily structural disease demonstrable on an imaging study.

Now, describe any consistent focal slowing, theta or delta, that indicates localized cerebral pathology. The focality may be present in a setting of a slow disorganized background, or may stand out against a relatively normal background. Finally, describe any bifrontal delta activity, its symmetry or asymmetry, rhythmicity, and amount.

After determining what the background of the record contains in terms of slowing, evaluate the presence or absence of epileptiform activity. Describe the type and location of any spikes, sharp waves, spike-wave complexes, or other paroxysmal discharges (e.g. episodic sharp theta or delta frequencies, including FIRDA). A statement concerning discharge abundance should be made. Focal discharges such as spikes may be obvious, or hidden in the ongoing background. Reliance on fairly strict definitions of epileptiform discharges is essential. Sometimes, the record seems to contain sharp potentials everywhere! Careful analysis will reveal that most of these putative sharp waves are simply the result of a polyrhythmic background – superimposition of various frequencies.

The alert recording having been assessed, now turn to the recording during drowsiness. In most cases, subjects become drowsy during some part of the record. Look for various drowsy patterns that are found in normal adult subjects. These include, but are not limited to, slowing of the PDR, interruption of the PDR by slower activities, anterior spread of a slowed PDR, generalized reduction in amplitude, appearance or increase in diffuse theta activity, bifrontal delta activity in older subjects, and generalized rhythmic 4 to 5 Hz activity in children. Note that subjects may drift in and out of drowsiness rapidly. This cannot be determined by clinical observation. Also look for roving eye movements in the anterior derivations; this is a good sign of drowsiness. There are relatively low-voltage slow potentials, maximal in the frontal regions. Vertex sharp waves may be seen during drowsiness and do not define entry into Stage II sleep. In addition, early sleep spindles may appear, usually less than 1 second in duration. POSTS and K-complexes may also appear without full development. These features, however, herald the approach of Stage II sleep.

**Important concept**: Recording of drowsiness is an essential element in EEG diagnosis. Often, pathological findings occur mainly, or only, during this state. Of particular importance is the precipitation, or exaggeration, of epileptiform activity (spikes, spike-wave complexes – also sharp waves if a broad definition is accepted). Slow wave abnormalities are frequently exaggerated during drowsiness. Bifrontal rhythmic delta (FIRDA) may become more prominent during this state. In any case, indicate the effect of drowsiness on the major findings.

After drowsiness, move to the main phenomena of sleep. Describe the features of Stage II sleep (established sleep spindles, vertex sharp waves, K-complexes, POSTS, and increased diffuse slowing in theta and delta ranges). At first, theta predominates, followed by increasing amounts of delta. Note that vertex sharp waves are not always sharp. On the other hand, they may be very sharp, and resemble spike potentials. In addition, they may be isolated and sporadic, or highly rhythmic.

Stage II sleep is followed by SWS. During this state the background is dominated by delta activity. At the same time, sleep spindles become less prominent and may disappear. In general, SWS is infrequently recorded in adults during routine EEG recording. On the other hand, SWS occurs frequently in young children, especially after they have been sedated. Include in your description the effect of sleep on any abnormalities previously noted – or new abnormalities that may appear.

You are now ready to dictate your report. Bear in mind always that you are trying to convey what patterns you have seen, what they mean, and how you can assist the clinician.

# APPENDIX

## INFLUENCE OF COMMON DRUGS ON THE EEG

Many common medications have effects on the brain, and thus on the EEG. Although these effects are not specific, it is important for our readers to be familiar with them in order to avoid an erroneous diagnosis of intrinsic brain pathology. A comprehensive review of this topic is beyond the scope of this book. We will discuss some of the common drugs you are likely to encounter along with their main effects on the recording.

### Barbiturates

Barbiturates produce an increase in the amount and amplitude of beta activity. The beta may reach high amplitudes and, although diffuse, is often most prominent in the frontal regions. As the blood level of the barbiturate rises, slower activities begin to invade the recording along with slowing of the posterior dominant rhythm. Barbiturate intoxication leads to changes similar to those associated with general anesthesia. Diffuse, unreactive delta activity may be recorded, while beta activity disappears. Later stages lead to burst-suppression and ultimately an isopotential or flat record. Abrupt withdrawal after long-term treatment may lead to asynchronous slowing along with generalized epileptiform activity.

### Benzodiazepines

Like barbiturates, benzodiazepines produce prominent beta activity. Even after the last dose of one of these drugs, excessive beta may persist for some days. Some diffuse theta range slowing may be seen along with attenuation of the posterior dominant rhythm. Paroxysmal synchronous slowing may be seen after long-term use. Effects of toxic doses are similar to those produced by other CNS depressants and correlate with the degree of mental status depression.

## Typical and atypical neuroleptics

Phenothiazines, thioxanthenes, and butyrophenones at therapeutic doses cause slowing of the PDR along with diffuse slow waves. They also may activate generalized paroxysmal slowing and sharp waves. In epileptic patients, phenothiazines may increase seizure frequency. The atypical neuroleptic, clozapine, produces an increase in diffuse slowing. Chronic use may lead to paroxysmal slowing with spikes or sharp waves. Risperidone, on the other hand, seems to have very little effect on the EEG.

## Lithium

Lithium may lead to diverse and prominent changes in the EEG. Although there is some correlation between the blood level of lithium and electrographic changes, there is considerable variability. One may see slowing of the PDR along with an increase in diffuse slowing. Intermittent rhythmic delta waves, most prominent in the frontal or occipital regions may appear, and triphasic waves have been described. Occasional spikes and focal slowing should not be interpreted as evidence of a structural lesion. With lithium intoxication, EEG abnormalities are usually marked and include considerable diffuse slow waves, triphasic waves, and multifocal epileptiform discharges. These findings may linger for days after clinical manifestations of intoxication have resolved.

## Tricyclic antidepressants

Tricyclic antidepressants such as imipramine, amitriptyline, doxepin, desipramine, and nortriptyline usually increase the amount of beta activity as well as theta activity in the record. The frequency of the PDR is usually decreased. Paroxysmal slow waves or even spikes may be seen, even at therapeutic doses. In patients with epilepsy, seizure frequency could be increased. With high doses, seizures have been reported in patients without a history of epilepsy. Acute intoxication may produce widespread poorly reactive alpha-range activity and spikes.

Note that some of the newer generation of antidepressants can increase seizure liability. This appears to be particularly true of bupropion.

## Antiepileptic drugs

Phenytoin, unlike barbiturates and benzodiazepines, does not produce prominent beta activity. Rather, it tends to cause an increase in the degree of diffuse slow waves in the theta range. With chronic use there usually is a decline in the frequency of the PDR. At toxic levels, diffuse irregular delta activity may be recorded along with paroxysmal rhythmic slow waves.

Carbamazepine usually has little effect on the EEG at therapeutic levels. An increase in diffuse slowing may occur. Epileptiform activity is usually not materially altered, although an increase in focal spikes has been reported.

Valproic acid at therapeutic levels produces little or no change in the EEG background. Its principal effect is a reduction in generalized epileptiform discharges, particularly 3 Hz spike-wave discharges. At toxic levels, valproate may produce an encephalopathy characterized by lethargy with a recording dominated by diffuse delta waves. In this setting, rare cases of epilepsia partialis continua have been observed along with focal epileptiform activity. In such patients there is no evidence of a structural brain lesion.

As of this writing the influence of several of the newer anti-epileptic agents on the EEG has not been clearly established. Gabapentin appears to have little effect on the EEG background. Lamotrigine also does not materially affect the background but, similar to valproic acid, there is a decline in generalized spike-wave discharges.

## THE ROLE OF THE EEG IN DETERMINING ANTI-EPILEPTIC DRUG TREATMENT

The EEG plays a potentially useful role in selecting an appropriate AED. Although there may be sufficient information to make an informed decision based on the clinical picture, this can be misleading. For example, in cases of generalized tonic-clonic convulsions (GTCC) it is not necessarily obvious whether the seizures are primarily or secondarily generalized. Likewise, in patients with apparent absence seizures, the clinical differentiation from complex partial seizures may be difficult. In both these instances the EEG offers assistance.

In both circumstances there are usually generalized spike-wave discharges, and in both cases focal discharges may be recorded. Thus, in those with absence attacks, one should select an agent that might be considered as an "anti-spike-wave" AED such as valproate. Topiramate and lamotrigine are also considerations and are preferred by some (especially in women of child-bearing age). If the EEG picture and clinical evidence is diagnostic of simple absence epilepsy without concomitant major seizures, ethosuximide should be considered. If the EEG reveals a temporal spike focus in a patient with apparent absence or confusional states, the choice would be one of the "focal" agents, either one of the newer agents of which there are now several, or one of the older agents such as carbamazepine or phenytoin. If, on the other hand, the EEG is indeterminate – that is a decision cannot be made between a focal or generalized abnormality (the EEG might be normal), then selection of a broad-spectrum agent would be a rational choice (e.g. valproate, lamotrigine, topiramate).

## GUIDELINES FOR TREATMENT OF GENERALIZED CONVULSIVE STATUS EPILEPTICUS (GCSE)

### Overt GCSE

Generalized convulsive status must be treated promptly and with intravenous medications. Ideally, treatment of GCSE should be carried out during constant

EEG monitoring. We understand that this is not always possible, but would advise that every effort be made to have a portable EEG machine available for nights and weekends. For the treatment of status it is not necessary to apply individual electrodes (with collodion or paste). Residents and fellows can easily acquire such facility in the use of the Electrocap®, which can be applied and ready to go in a few minutes. With a little organization, the ability to record the EEG during status should be possible in many (if not most) instances.

Drawing on the results of a large multicenter study of the treatment of GCSE, with some modification, we recommend immediate administration of lorazepam (0.1 mg/kg IV) at 1 mg/min followed by a loading dose of fosphenytoin (20 mg/kg phenytoin equivalents [PE] IV). If given early in the course of status, this combination has a good chance of success. Success is defined as elimination of all clinical and electrographic seizure activity. (Remember that elimination of clinical seizure activity is not evidence that status has truly resolved.)

The first treatment may not be successful. With the patient quiescent, the EEG may show continuing discharges (Treiman pattern II or III, for example), or perhaps an epileptic burst-suppression pattern – that is, the bursts contain spikes or sharp waves. If additional treatment is not given, the patient's clinical seizures are likely to recur, or the patient simply will not wake up. In the event of failure of lorazepam followed by fosphenytoin, the second drug we give is phenobarbital, 20 mg/kg IV at 50 mg/min. Residents have sometimes queried this course because of the sedative properties of phenobarbital. The point here, however, is suppression of status, accepting the side effects of the barbiturate. The truth is that phenobarbital is an excellent AED; in fact, it is used by some as a first drug in the treatment of status. In any event, the second treatment with phenobarbital may be effective in an additional 20 percent of cases. The two consecutive treatments should be administered within 1 hour.

If the second treatment fails, evidenced by continuing epileptiform activity in the EEG (Treiman stages II–V), we advise immediate resort to general anesthesia (GA). After failure of the first treatment, it is wise to inform an anesthesiologist that intubation may be required. Three modalities of GA are used in our institution, although there are others. The main principle of selection is experience in using the modality. Pentobarbital has a long record of effectiveness and often is selected. More recently, propofol has become popular, mainly because of its rapid elimination. This characteristic allows prompt assessment of the EEG for epileptiform activity and rapid reinstitution of GA if it persists. Midazolam also has a following. Comparative studies of these agents are not available. We do note, however, that some patients who do not respond adequately to one of these agents may do so when the treatment is changed.

### Subtle GCSE

Subtle GCSE presents a true diagnostic and therapeutic challenge. It is the job of the electroencephalographer to make the diagnosis and communicate immediately with the clinician, who may not realize that the patient is still in status. A note: subtle status can be treated effectively only under EEG control, inasmuch as there is no way to determine clinically whether or not status has been suppressed. In our experience, subtle status occurs most often in ICUs and other acute hospital units (e.g. transplant units). An EEG machine should be stationed at the patient's bedside while treatment is administered and during the post-treatment period. Fortunate readers will be able to take advantage of acute seizure units or ICUs wired for digital EEG transmission.

The treatment of subtle GCSE is similar to that of overt GCSE. The combination of lorazepam and fosphenytoin may be used as initial treatment, although an argument could be made for starting with phenobarbital. The latter drug proved marginally better than phenytoin in the Veterans Affairs study of status, but the difference was not statistically significant. Many would prefer to start with the relatively non-sedating phenytoin (fosphenytoin), bearing in mind that the benzodiazepines are also markedly sedating. In any event, subtle status will usually require more than one treatment. Even then, the ictal activity is difficult to suppress. Thus, many such patients will require general anesthesia. As in overt GCSE, hypotension is a major problem. Again, the electroencephalographer is the point person in treating this form of status, working closely with the clinician. He or she must ensure that all epileptiform activity is eradicated (including spikes as part of a burst-suppression pattern), as rapidly as possible, commensurate with maintaining cardiovascular stability. In most cases, however, pressors will be required.

## GUIDELINES FOR TREATMENT OF NON-CONVULSIVE STATUS EPILEPTICUS (NCSE)

Treatment of NCSE differs from that of GCSE in that urgency is somewhat diminished. That is not to say that NCSE should not be treated promptly with adequate doses of AEDs. This is particularly true in patients in NCSE who have marked impairment of consciousness. Bear in mind the wide variation in the clinical manifestations of NCSE. Indeed, patients with NCSE characterized by mild confusion, or even personality change, may continue in these states for days, weeks, or even months. After treatment, most such individuals appear to have sustained no obvious lasting neurological deficit.

Patients who develop NCSE in the context of systemic illness require urgent treatment, inasmuch as the associated status impairs overall recovery. By the same token, the underlying unstable medical or neurological condition impairs the ability to suppress status. It is important, however, to be aware that overtreatment may result in worsening of a patient's already precarious condition. Thus, each patient's clinical status must be carefully evaluated and the therapy individualized.

### Absence NCSE

Treatment of absence NCSE with synchronous spike-wave discharges is relatively easy, and outcome is generally excellent. Ideally, treatment should be administered under EEG control and should be intravenous. A benzodiazepine, preferably lorazepam because of its longer duration of action, is effective in most cases. One may begin with a relatively low dose (compared to treatment of GCSE), say 2 mg in older children, followed by another 2 mg if the response is incomplete. In younger children the dose should be adjusted downward. Intravenous valproate is also effective, administering 1000 mg in divided doses (less in younger children). In the latter case valproate may be continued orally, adjusting the dose if the patient already was receiving the drug.

### Complex Partial NCSE (CP-NCSE)

There is no unanimity of opinion concerning the treatment of complex partial NCSE (CP-NCSE). Lorazepam is effective in many cases, possibly more so in those with NCSE secondary to drug withdrawal. A strong case can also be made for the use of valproate in view of the synchronous ictal discharges. Others advocate treatment with phenytoin or fosphenytoin because the status in reality has a focal onset, even though not evident on the EEG. The authors advocate the use of IV lorazepam in most cases, followed by fosphenytoin. In the elderly it is important to treat incrementally. We have had some success in older subjects by starting with 0.5 to 1.0 mg IV. The trick is to use only enough medication to suppress the discharges without putting the patient to sleep. We are successful in only a small percentage, however. Treating with additional doses should follow if there is no effect. In older adults, we usually do not go above 2 to 3 mg before crossing over to fosphenytoin.

As with GCSE, CP-NCSE should be treated under EEG control whenever possible. The electroencephalographer looks for disappearance of ictal activity that, in many cases, will be replaced with sleep patterns. In addition, when synchronous discharges are suppressed, focal abnormalities may be revealed.

**Note**: CP-NCSE, while often quite obvious from an EEG point of view, may have relatively subtle electrographic manifestations. Patients demonstrating with rhythmic or quasi-rhythmic sharply contoured delta activity in the frontal regions are easily misdiagnosed by the unwary or inexperienced. Thus, the electroencephalographer's input, and indeed presence, is a critical factor in successful treatment.

## CEREBRAL DEATH RECORDING

For many years the EEG has been the mainstay for a declaration of cerebral death. More recently, however, many jurisdictions have discarded the EEG in favor of two thorough neurological examinations, made 12 to 24 hours apart, that demonstrate absence of cerebral and brainstem function. Nonetheless, some clinicians wish to obtain an EEG in addition to the clinical examinations. Whereas a routine record that demonstrates severe depression of cerebral activity (say, in the context of anoxic damage) at normal sensitivity settings implies a poor prognosis, it is not considered adequate to make an electrographic diagnosis of cerebral death (electrocerebral silence, ECS). In order to maximize the chance of recording low voltage potentials that are not evident on routine recording, special recording guidelines for obtaining an EEG in patients suspected on clinical grounds of sustaining cerebral death have been developed by the American Electroencephalographic Society. The technologist must pay meticulous attention to detail when carrying out an ECS recording. Minimum requirements include:

1. Placement of at least eight scalp electrodes.
2. Interelectrode distance of at least 10 cm. For example, with A-P bipolar recording, skipping electrodes (e.g. Fp1 → T3; T3 → O1) might be used, covering temporal and paracentral chains.
3. Interelectrode impedance between 100 and 10,000 Ohms.
4. Integrity of the entire recording system should be tested.
5. Recording at a sensitivity of 2 μV.
6. Recording for at least 30 minutes.
7. Recording with the high-frequency (HF) filter not set below 30 Hz, and the low-frequency (LF) filter set not above 1 Hz.
8. Demonstrable non-reactivity to somatosensory (painful), visual (e.g. photic stimulation), and auditory stimuli.

EKG and EOG leads are also employed. Other requirements must also be met. The patient's temperature must be above 35°C. The patient must not be receiving drugs that might depress cortical function (e.g. barbiturates, benzodiazepines). If there is doubt, obtain serum levels.

A declaration of ECS rests on the absence of discernible electrocortical potentials under the above conditions. This is dependent on obtaining a relatively artifact-free recording. The accepted standard is that potentials up to 2 μV are permitted (considered the limit of so-called machine "noise"). The reader should be able to identify any other potentials as clearly artifactual in nature (e.g. electrode, ECG, artifacts due to any movement around the recording area). The technician must note any observations that relate to presumed artifacts.

As mentioned, criteria for a declaration of cerebral death vary. With respect to the EEG, some jurisdictions may still require two EEGs recorded 12 to 24 hours apart and demonstrating ECS, in addition to clinical examinations. Others may require a single EEG at the time of a second neurological examination. Still others may not require an EEG at all, and rely on clinical criteria. The reader is advised to check local legal and institutional requirements.

# GLOSSARY

**Alpha.** Rhythmic, sinusoidal frequency at 8 to 13 Hz, most prominent in the occipital derivations. Recorded in waking, resting state. Symmetrical, or higher in voltage over non-dominant hemisphere. Attenuates with eye-opening or mental activity.

**Asynchrony.** The opposite of synchrony – that is, the independent or non-simultaneous occurrence of EEG waves over the two hemispheres.

**Alpha coma.** Infrequently seen after a catastrophic brain injury such as anoxia. The patient is comatose, and the EEG shows alpha range activity in widespread distribution, usually maximal in the frontal regions. There is no reactivity as seen with the alpha rhythm. Prognosis is poor.

**Alpha variants.** Rhythmic frequencies related harmonically to the alpha. Slow alpha variant is half the alpha frequency; fast alpha variant twice. May coexist with alpha or appear alone. Notched appearance of slow alpha variant gives clue to its presence.

**Attenuation.** Reduction of EEG activity. An example is reduction or disappearance of the alpha following eye opening.

**Background.** The underlying activity of the brain. Focal slow waves, synchronous bifrontal slowing, or epileptiform discharges are said to interrupt the background. Not synonymous with the alpha that itself is seen against the background.

**Band.** Refers to a frequency range. For example, the alpha lies in the 8 to 13 Hz frequency band.

**Beta.** Rhythmic, usually low voltage activity at 14 Hz or greater. Usually maximal over the fronto-central regions. Increases in amplitude and becomes more widespread with certain drugs.

**BETS.** Benign epileptiform transients of sleep, also known as small sharp spikes (SSS). Positive spike potentials appearing in the temporal regions. Of no clinical significance.

**Bilateral synchrony.** Refers to waveforms appearing simultaneously over both hemispheres, often applied to generalized spike-wave complexes (e.g. as seen in simple absence attacks).

**Bipolar recording.** Method of recording wherein the activity picked up by a particular electrode (say, a spike discharge) is conducted to opposite sides of adjacent amplifiers. In one amplifier the input is in Lead I with a resulting upward deflection of the display or write-out. In the adjacent amplifier the input is in Lead II with a resultant downward deflection. This creates the phase reversal.

**Bisynchronous.** Occurring simultaneously in the two hemispheres. Really the same as synchronous (which is preferred).

**Blocking.** The same as attenuation; for example, the alpha is blocked with eye opening. Also used to describe an amplifier's response to a temporary voltage overload during which there are wide excursions of the write out or display preempting recording of EEG activity.

**Breach rhythm.** Team referring to localized increased amplitude of background rhythms that result from an underlying craniotomy or other rent in the calvarium. (Breach: a broken or torn place. *Webster's World College Dictionary,* 4th Edn.) Beta activity with admixed slower frequencies may appear quite sharp and should not be mistaken for epileptiform discharges.

**Build-up.** Used to describe the high-voltage, synchronous slow wave response during hyperventilation.

**Burst-suppression.** Episodic or paroxysmal potentials, slow or sharp, or a combination of both, followed by suppression of cerebral activity. Suppressions vary widely in duration.

**Calibration.** Display of a square wave signal injected into the amplifiers, measured in microvolts/cm or mm. Demonstrates the response of the system to particular voltages.

**Channel.** Refers to the output of an amplifier that displays electrical information. The number of channels displayed by an EEG apparatus varies, but often is on the order of 20.

**Common average reference recording.** Referential recording in which the activity from the exploring electrode is compared to the averaged activity of the remaining electrodes on the scalp.

**Common mode rejection.** Characteristic of differential amplification where a signal that is the same in the two amplifier inputs is "rejected," or not recorded (there is no potential difference).

**Common mode signal.** Any activity, either physiological or environmental, that is the same at the two inputs of an amplifier.

**Complex.** A description of time-locked frequencies, usually applied to epileptiform activity. The best example is the spike-wave complex in which each discharge has the same temporal relationship of the spike to the following wave.

**Delta.** Waves in the 0.5 to 3.5 Hz frequency band. Not components of the normal, waking adult EEG with some exceptions.

**Depression.** Refers to reduction of amplitude or voltage due to a disease process, focal or generalized. An example would be the depression of amplitude sometimes recorded over a subdural hematoma or hygroma.

**Derivation.** Recording from an electrode pair with the output displayed in one channel of the recording.

**Differential amplifier.** An amplifier whose output is proportional to the difference in voltage between the two input terminals.

**Diffuse.** Occurring generally over the two hemispheres, usually used to describe slowing. Contrast with focal slowing.

**Discharge.** Used to describe a paroxysmal event (e.g. a spike), or electrographic ictal activity (e.g. a new paroxysmal rhythmic frequency).

**Electrode impedance.** Opposition to AC current flow between an electrode and its interface with the scalp. Measured between pairs of electrodes and measured in Ohms (thousands of Ohms in EEG work). It is important that electrode impedances are generally equal and relatively low in order to ensure good, artifact-free recording.

**Electrographic seizure.** Recorded ictal activity with or without clinical accompaniment. May be focal with recruiting rhythms, or generalized.

**Epileptiform discharges.** Refers to spikes and spike-wave complexes. Sharp waves are sometimes included. Any paroxysmal rhythmic frequency (e.g. beta, alpha, or even delta) may also be classified as epileptiform.

**Equipotential.** Term used to indicate equal potentials at different electrodes.

**Exploring electrode.** The designation of an electrode that records cerebral activity of interest.

**Extreme spindles.** Very high-voltage sleep spindles sometimes found in mental retardation.

**Fast activity.** Synonym for beta activity.

**FIRDA.** Frontal intermittent rhythmic delta activity. High-voltage bifrontal rhythmic waves at about 3 Hz, indicative of deep midline lesions. Also seen in acute hydrocephalus or frontal lesions. May be asymmetric.

**Filters.** Particular circuits within amplifiers that attenuate either high or low frequencies.

**Focus.** Refers to the location of maximal potential.

**Fourteen and six positive spikes (14/6).** Electropositive spikes at 14 or 6 Hz, or a combination of both. Usually maximal in the posterior temporal derivations and best recorded with wide interelectrode distances (e.g. the crossed ear reference). Of doubtful clinical significance.

**High-frequency filter.** Reduces the sensitivity of the EEG to high frequencies. Can be adjusted by a stepped control available on all EEG machines and digital reading stations.

**High-pass filter.** Synonym for low-frequency filter.

**Hyperventilation.** Standard procedure during routine EEG recording. The subject is asked to overbreathe deeply as a faster than normal rate for a period of 3 to 5 minutes. Often activates latent or minor abnormalities, especially spike-wave discharges.

**Hypsarrhythmia.** Chaotic, very high-voltage discharges consisting of an admixture of generalized spikes, sharp waves and slow waves, characteristic of infantile spasms. One may also see focal discharges as well as intermittent suppressions of cerebral activity.

**Input I.** Refers to the first of two inputs to an amplifier (Lead 1 – in the UK, the black lead).

**Input II.** Refers to the second of two inputs to an amplifier (Lead 2 – in the UK, the white lead).

**Interelectrode distance.** Distance between pairs of electrodes.

**Isolated.** Refers to a waveform, for example a spike or slow wave, occurring as an individual, non-repetitive event.

**Isopotentiality.** Term used for lack of electrocortical potentials. Seen after severe cerebral damage secondary to cardiopulmonary arrest, or during deep anesthesia. Sometimes referred to as "flat line."

**K-Complexes.** High-voltage mono- or multiphasic paroxysmal slow potentials with trailing sleep spindles. Prominent during State II sleep, but may occur during waking and drowsiness in response to external stimulus (alerting response).

**Lambda waves.** Electropositive sharp potentials recorded in the occipital regions, generated when a subject is exploring the environment.

**Lateralized.** Used to indicate activities that are recorded in both hemispheres but are more prominent, of higher amplitude, more frequent, or of higher amplitude on one side.

**Lead.** Refers to an electrode and its connection to the EEG machine.

**Low frequency filter.** Reduces the sensitivity of the EEG to low frequencies. Can be adjusted by a stepped control available on all EEG machines and digital reading stations.

**Low-pass filter.** Synonym for high-frequency filter.

**Mittens.** Episodic slow potentials with associated blunted sharp component. Recorded in the frontal regions during State II sleep. Mittens have no clinical significance and must be differentiated from epileptiform discharges.

**Montage.** Term used to indicate the pattern of display of EEG activity.

**Nasopharyngeal electrode.** Relatively thin, insulated wire with an exposed tip, introduced through the nose, coming to rest at the back of the nasopharynx adjacent to the sphenoid bone. Records activity from the inferomesial temporal lobe. Used less frequently today due to unavoidable artifacts (pulse, breathing, swallowing) and its discomfort.

**Noise.** Small currents in an EEG channel related to the machine circuitry, not physiological potentials.

**Notch filter.** A circuit that filters out a narrow band of frequencies, for example a 60 (50) Hz signal. Particularly important when recording in ICU settings where a variety of electrical equipment is in use.

**Mu rhythm.** Sometimes referred to as wicket rhythm. Mu rhythm is a normal finding. It appears as sharply contoured rhythmic waves at 7 to 11 Hz, maximal over the central regions. May be unilateral or bilateral. Responds to movement of the opposite upper extremity (e.g. making a fist), or thinking about it.

**OIRDA.** Occipital Intermittent Rhythmic Delta Activity. Rhythmic waves occurring in the occipital regions, indicative of deep occipital lesions.

**Organization.** Refers to a comparison of an EEG to recognized normal patterns. For example, a well-organized adult waking EEG usually contains regular alpha rhythm in the occipital regions, beta activity in the fronto-central regions, and little else. If the alpha is disrupted by slower frequencies, the record might be said to be somewhat disorganized. If there is no posterior dominant rhythm along with a great deal of generalized delta range slowing, the record might be said to be completely disorganized and slow.

**Parodoxical alpha.** Alpha rhythm that appears after eye opening, seen in drowsy subjects (the opposite of what happens in alert subjects).

**Paroxysm.** Term used to indicate a waveform that arises suddenly from the background, for example a spike discharge.

**Pattern.** A characteristic EEG activity, for example 3 Hz spike-wave discharge or triphasic waves.

**PEDs.** Periodic Epileptiform Discharges. Generalized epileptiform discharges, often occurring in the context of generalized convulsive status epilepticus of the subtle type.

**Periodicity.** Refers to recurrent focal or generalized discharges with a relatively fixed interdischarge interval (the period).

**Phantom spike-wave.** A normal variant characterized by low-voltage 6 Hz spike wave discharges.

**Phase Reversal.** Localization principle of bipolar recording. The electrical phenomenon of interest (e.g. a slow wave or spike) point toward each other in adjacent channels.

**Photic driving (also known as the following response).** Response to intermittent photic stimulation recorded in the occipital regions. The evoked waves are time-locked to the flash rate. If there is a 1:1 response, it is termed the fundamental. If the response is twice the flash frequency it is termed a harmonic response, and if half the frequency it is termed the subharmonic. All are normal.

**Photomyoclonic response.** Response to intermittent photic stimulation consisting of repetitive muscle action potentials, maximal in the frontal derivations, linked to the flash frequency. The response ceases when the flash train stops.

**Photoparoxysmal Response.** Generalized, synchronous epileptiform activity consisting of spike and poly-spike wave complexes, maximal in the frontal regions, evoked by intermittent photic stimulation. When recorded, the technician must stop the flash stimulus immediately to avoid the possibility of precipitating a generalized seizure. The response usually outlasts cessation of the flash train by 1 or 2 seconds. Also known as the photoconvulsive response.

**Photosensitivity.** General term in denoting an abnormal response to intermittent photic stimulation including the photoparoxysmal response. With lesser degrees of photosensitivity, occipital spikes or less generalized spikes or sharp waves are time-linked to the flash frequency. The response stops when the flash train ceases.

**PLEDs.** Periodic lateralized epileptiform discharges. Periodic epileptiform potentials, confined to one hemisphere, occurring adjacent to an area of cerebral infarction or tumor.

**POSTS.** Positive occipital sharp transients of sleep. Electropositive sharp potentials, maximal in occipital derivations. May be quite prominent. Often noted during State II sleep. May occur in rhythmic runs. Formally known as lambdoidal waves.

**Projected rhythms.** Waves recorded at a distance from the recording electrodes, usually subcortical. FIRDA is an example (q.v.). Also known as rhythms at a distance.

**Reactivity.** Alteration of EEG activity by external sensory stimulation. In a comatose patient, usually a favorable sign.

**Reference electrode.** Electrode placed in various locations, for example an ear or at the vertex. In referential recording the activity from an exploring electrode is compared to the reference (potential difference). Activity from the reference electrode is conducted to Lead II of an amplifier.

**Rhythmic temporal theta.** Normal variant. Rhythmic 4 to 7 Hz waves in the temporal regions, recorded during drowsiness. May be notched in appearance. Formerly known as psychomotor variant.

**Sensitivity.** Ratio of input voltage to output recorded in a channel of the EEG recording.

**Sharp-slow complex.** Epileptiform pattern consisting of a sharp wave followed by a slow wave, usually in the delta frequency band. A typical example is the generalized sharp-slow complex at 2 Hz, typical of the Lennox–Gastaut syndrome.

**Sharp wave.** Paroxysmal sharp potential with duration of 80 to 200 ms. Because of longer duration, less sharp than a spike, but similar in configuration.

**Sleep Spindles.** Rhythmic, sometimes spindle-shaped activity at 12 to 14 Hz (± 2), indicative of Stage II sleep. Usually maximal over central or frontocentral regions. Formally called sigma rhythm.

**Slowing.** Activities slower than alpha activity.

**Sphenoidal electrodes.** Insulated electrode wires with an exposed tip, introduced through the mandibular notch via a hollow needle. After the needle comes to rest near the foramen ovale the needle is withdrawn. Records activity from the inferomesial temporal lobe.

**Spike.** Paroxysmal sharp potential with duration of 20 to 80 msec. More rapid rise than fall time; often followed by low-voltage slow potential.

**Spike-wave complex.** Spike followed by time-linked, high-voltage slow wave. Various frequency bands (typically 3–5 Hz). Synchronous, rhythmic 3 Hz spike-wave runs typical of simple absence attacks. Synchronous 4 to 5 Hz spike-wave runs seen in primary generalized epilepsy with generalized convulsions. Irregular rapid spike-wave discharges are typical of juvenile myoclonic epilepsy (JME). See also sharp-slow complex.

**Spread.** Activity spreading out from its site of origin – for example alpha activity that is represented anterior to the occipital regions.

**SREDA.** Subclinical rhythmic electroencephalographic discharges of adults. A normal variant. Resembles focal electrographic seizure activity in a temporal region, but there is no recruiting and no clinical manifestations.

**Theta.** Waves in the 4 to 7 Hz frequency band. May be a normal finding or may indicate pathology. Some theta is acceptable in the normal waking adult EEG.

**TIRDA.** Temporal Intermittent Rhythmic Delta Activity. Rhythmic waves occurring in the temporal regions, indicative of deep temporal lesions.

**Trace alternant.** Normal pattern found in newborns characterized by bursts of slowing, perhaps with sharp potentials, alternating with periods of low voltage.

**Transient.** Similar to paroxysm. A wave that suddenly interrupts the background.

**Triphasic wave.** Paroxysmal potential associated with hepatic encephalopathy, or other metabolic encephalopathies. Quite sharp in configuration with three phases (sometimes two), synchronous, maximum bifrontally. May be mistaken for epileptiform activity.

**Youth Waves.** Sharply contoured delta waves underlying the posterior dominant rhythm. Sometimes called posterior temporo-occipital slow waves of youth. This activity is prominent in childhood and adolescence. Youth waves attenuate with eye opening and are thought to be generated at thalamic levels, dependent on thalamocortical pathways.

**Vertex sharp waves.** Recorded during Stage II sleep, but also noted during late drowsiness. May reach high-voltage. Isolated or repetitive. Sometimes as sharp as spikes. Usually maximal in central regions.

# REFERENCES

## EEG TEXTBOOKS

Barlow, John S. *The Electroencephalogram*. MIT Press, 1993.

Blume, Warren T, Kaibara, Masako, Young, G Brian. *Atlas of Adult Electroencephalography*. Lippincott Williams & Williams, 2001.

Clancy, RR, Chung, HL, Temple, JP. *Atlas of Electroencephalography*, Volume 1. Elsevier Science, 1999.

Daly, David K, Klass, Donald W (eds). *Current Practice of Electroencephalography*. Raven, 1979

Fisch, Bruce J. *Fish and Spehlmann's EEG Primer*. 3rd edition. Elsevier Science, 1999.

Hughes, John R. *EEG in Clinical Practice*. 2nd edition. Butterworth–Heinemann Medical, 1994.

Lueders, Hans, Noachtar, Soheyl, Benson, Judy K. (Translator), Ross, Allan (ed.). *Atlas and Classification of Electroencephalography*. WB Saunders Co., 2000.

Niedermeyer, Ernst (ed.), Loopes Da Silva, Fernando (eds.). *Electroencephalography: Basic Principles, Clinical Applications, and Related Fields*. 4th edition. Williams & Wilkins, 1999.

Sperling, Michael R, Morrell, Martha J. *Atlas of Electroencephalography*, Volume 2. Elsevier Science, 1999.

Sperling, Michael R. *Atlas of Electroencephalography*, Volume 3. Elsevier Science, 1999.

## TEXTS OUT OF PRINT BUT WORTH SEEKING OUT

Binnie CD, Rowan AJ, Gutter Th. *A Manual of Electroencephalographic Technology*. Cambridge, University Press, 1982.

Gibbs FA, Gibbs EL. *Atlas of Electroencephalography*, Volume 1. Cambridge MA, Addison-Wesley, 1950.

Gibbs FA, Gibbs EL. *Atlas of Electroencephalography*, Volume 2. *Epilepsy*. Reading MA, Addison-Wesley, 1952.

Hill JDN, Parr G. *Electroencephalography*. London, MacDonald, 2nd edition, 1963. (An old war-horse, but fun for classic references.)

Kiloh LG, McComas AJ, Osselton JW. *Clinical Electroencephalography*. London, Butterworths, 1972.

Klass DW, Daly DD. *Current Practice of Clinical Electroencephalography*. New York, Raven, 1979.

Kooi KA, Tucker RP, Narstakk RE. *Fundamentals of Electroencephalography*. Hagerstown, Harper and Row, 1978.

Scott DF. *Understanding EEG*. London, Duckworth, 1976.

## ARTICLES AND CHAPTERS

### Chapter 1: Origin and Technical Aspects of the EEG

#### *Origin of the EEG*

Adrian ED, Matthews BHC. The Berger rhythm: potential changes from the occipital lobes in man. *Brain* 1934;**57**:536–385.

Andesen P, Andersson SA. *Physiological Basis of the Alpha Rhythm*. 1968: New York, Appleton.

Berger H. Ueber das elektroenkephalogramm des menschen. *Arch Psychiatr* 1929;**87**:527–570.

Buzsaki G, Traub R. Physiological basis of EEG activity. In: J Engel Jr, TA Pedley (eds), *Epilepsy: A Comprehensive Textbook*. Philadelphia: Lippincott-Raven, 1997:819–830.

Creutzfeldt O, Houchin J. Section I. Neuronal basis of EEG-waves. In: A Remond (ed.), *Handbook of Electroencephalography and Clinical Neurophysiology*, Volume 2C. Amsterdam: Elsevier, 1974;5–55.

Dempsey EW, Morison RS. The production of rhythmically recurrent cortical potentials after localized thalamic stimulation. *Am J Physiol* 1942;**135**:293–300.

Goldensohn ES. Neurophysiological substrates of EEG activity. In: D Klass, D Daly (eds), *Current Practice of Clinical Neurophysiology*. New York: Raven, 1979;421–440.

Moruzzi G, Magoun HW. Brain stem reticular formation and activation of the EEG. *Electroenceph Clin Neurophysiol* 1949;**1**:455–473.

#### *Technical Considerations*

American EEG Society Guidelines in EEG, 1-7 (Revised 1985). *J Clin Neurophysiol* 1985;**3**: 131–168.

Binnie CD. Recording techniques: montages, electrodes, amplifiers and filters. In: AM Halliday, SR Butler, R Paul (eds) *A Textbook of Clinical Neurophysiology*. New York: John Wiley, 1987;3–22.

Binnie CD, Rowan AJ, Gutter Th. *A Manual of Electroencephalographic Technology*. Cambridge: University Press, 1982.

Butler, R Paul (eds), *A Textbook of Clinical Neurophysiology*. Chichester, 1987, Wiley, 3–22.

Goldman D. The clinical use of the "average" reference electrode in monopolar recording. *Electroenceph Clin Neurophysiol* 1950;**2**:211–214.

Homan RW, Herman J, Purdy P. Cerebral localization of international 10-20 system electrode placement. *Electroenceph Clin Neurophysiol* 1987;**55**:376–382.

Jasper HH. Report of the committee on methods of clinical examination in electroencephalography. *Electroenceph Clin Neurophysiol* 1958;**10**:370–375.

Jasper HH. The ten-twenty electrode system of the International Federation. *Electroenceph Clin Neurophysiol* 1958;**10**:371–375.

Klass DW. Symposium on EEG montages: which, when, why and whither. Introduction. *Am J EEG Technol* 1977;**17**:1–3.

Lesser RP, Lueders H, Dinner DS, Morris H. An introduction to the basic concepts of polarity and localization. *J Clin Neurophysiol* 1985;**2**:45–61.

Silverman D. The anterior temporal electrode and the ten-twenty system. *Electroenceph Clin Neurophysiol* 1960;**12**:735–737.

## *Artifacts*

Beaussart M, Guiev JD. Section III. Artefacts. In: A Remond (ed.), *Handbook of Electroencephalography and Clinical Neurophysiology*, Volume 11A. Amsterdam: Elsevier, 1977;80–96.

Brittenham D. Recognition and reduction of physiological artifacts. *Am J EEG Technol* 1974;**14**:158–165.

Saunders MF. Artifacts: activity of noncerebral origin in the EEG. In: DW Klass, DD Daly (eds), *Current Practice of Clinical Electroencephalography*. New York: Raven Press, 1979;37–68.

Stones EA, Whitehead MK, MacGillivray BB. The nature of the eye blink artefact. *Proc Electrophysiol Technol Assoc* 1967;**14**:208–214.

Westmoreland BF, Espinosa RE, Klass DW. Significant prosopo-glossopharyngeal movements affecting the electroencephalogram. *Am J EEG Technol* 1973;**13**:59–70.

## Chapter 2: The Normal EEG

### *The Normal Adult EEG*

Chatrian GE, Lairy GC (eds). Part A. The EEG of the waking adult. In: A Remond (ed.), *Handbook of Electroencephalopathy and Clinical Neurophysiology*, Volume 6A. Amsterdam: Elsevier, 1976.

Dement W, Kleitman N. Cyclic variations in EEG during sleep and their relation to eye movements, body mobility, and dreaming. *Electroenceph Clin Neurophysiol* 1957; **9**:673–690.

Erwin CW, Sommerville ER, Radtke RA. A review of electroencephalographic features of normal sleep. *J Clin Neurophysiol* 1984;**1**:253–274.

Hughes JR, Cayaffa JJ. The EEG in patients at different ages without organic cerebral disease. *Electroenceph Clin Neurophysiol* 1977;**42**:776–784.

Hughes JR. Normal limits in the EEG. In: AM Halliday, SR Butler, R Paul (eds), *A Textbook of Clinical Neurophysiology* Chichester: Wiley, 1987;105–154.

Kozelka JW, Pedley TA. Beta and mu rhythms. *J Clin Neurophysiol* 1990;**7**:191–208.

Markand O. Alpha rhythms. *J Clin Neurophysiol* 1990;**7**:163–190.

Rechtschaffen A, Kales A. A Manual of Standardized Terminology, Techniques and Scoring System for Sleep Stages of Human Subjects. Washington, DC, US Government Printing Office, NIH Publications no. 204, 1968.

Schachter SC, Ito M, Wannamaker BB, Rak I, Ruggles K, Matsuo F, Wilner A, Jacker R, Gilliam F, Morris G, Skantz J, Sperling M, Buchhalter J, Drislane FW, Ives J, Schomer DL. Incidence of spikes and paroxysmal rhythmic events in overnight ambulatory computer-assisted EEGs of normal subjects: a multicenter study. *J Clin Neurophysiol* 1998;**15**:251–255.

Westmoreland B. Normal and benign EEG patterns. *Am J EEG Technol* 1982;**22**:3–31.

### *Special Considerations in Children*

Blum WT. *Atlas of Pediatric EEG*. New York: Raven, 1982.

Eeg-Olofsson O. The development of the electroencephalogram in normal adolescents from the age of 16 through 21 years. *Neuropaediatrie* 1971;**3**:11–45.

Petersen I, Eeg-Olofsson O. The development of the electroencephalogram in normal children from the age of 1 through 15 years. Nonparoxysmal activity. *Neuropaediatrie* 1971;**2**: 247–304.

Tharp BR. Neonatal and pediatric electroencephalography. In: MJ Aminoff (ed.), *Electrodiagnosis in Clinical Neurology.* New York: Churchill-Livingstone, 1980;67–117.

Westmoreland BF, Klass DW. Electroencephalography: Electroencephalograms of neonates, infants and children. In: J Daube (ed.), *Clinical Neurophysiology.* Philadelphia: FA Davis, 1996;104–113.

## Special Considerations in the Elderly

Arenal AM, Brenner RP, Reynolds CF. Temporal slowing in the elderly revisited. *Am J EEG Technol* 1986;**26**:105–114.

Hubbard O, Sunde D, Goldensohn ES. The EEG in centenarians. *Electroenceph Clin Neurophysiol* 1976;**40**:407–417.

Katz RI, Horowitz GR. Electroencephalogram in the septuagenarian: Studies in a normal geriatric population. *J Am Geriatr Soc* 1982;**30**:273–275.

Klass DW, Brenner RP. Electroencephalography of the elderly. *J Clin Neurophysiol* 1995;**27**:43–47.

Lee KS, Pedley TA. Electroencephalography and seizures in the elderly. In: AJ Rowan, RE Ramsay (eds), *Seizures and Epilepsy in the Elderly.* Boston: Butterworth–Heinemann, 1997;139–158.

Niedermeyer E. EEG and old age. In: E Niedermeyer, F Lopes da Silva (eds), *Electroencephalography: Basic Principles, Clinical Applications and Related Fields.* Baltimore: Williams and Wilkins, 1993;301–308.

Oken BS, Kaye JA. Electrophysiologic function in the healthy extremely old. *Neurology* 1992;**42**:519–526.

Torres F, Faoro A, Loewenson R, Johnson E. The electroencephalogram of elderly subjects revisited. *Electroenceph Clin Neurophysiol* 1983;**56**:391–398.

Visser SL, Hooijer C, Jonker C, Van Tilburg W, DeRijke W. Anterior temporal focal abnormalities in EEG in normal aged subjects: correlations with psychological and CT brain scan findings. *Electroenceph Clin Neurophysiol* 1987;**66**:1–7.

## Activation Procedures

Binnie CD, Coles PA, Margerison JH. The influence of end-tidal carbon dioxide tension on EEG changes during routine hyperventilation in different age groups. *Electroenceph Clin Neurophysiol* 1969;**27**:304–306.

Drury I. Activation procedures. In: E Wyllie (ed.), *The Treatment of Epilepsy. Principles and Practice,* 2nd edition. Baltimore: Williams and Wilkins, 1997;251–263.

Ellingson RJ, Wilken K, Bennett DR. Efficacy of sleep deprivation as an activation procedure in epilepsy patients. *J Clin Neurophysiol* 1984;**1**:83–102.

Fountain NB, Kim JS, Lee SI. Sleep deprivation activates epileptiform discharges independent of the activating effects of sleep. *J Clin Neurophysiol* 1998;**15**:69–75.

Gabor AJ, Seyal M. Effect of sleep on the electroencephalographic manifestations of epilepsy. *J Clin Neurophysiol* 1986;**3**:23–38.

Gloor P, Tsai C, Haddad F. An assessment of the value of sleep-electroencephalography for the diagnosis of temporal lobe epilepsy. *Electroenceph Clin Neurophysiol* 1958;**10**:633–648.

Heppenstall ME. The relation between the effects of the blood sugar levels and hyperventilation on the electroencephalogram. *J Neurol Neurosurg Psychiatr* 1944;**4**:112–118.

Hughes JR. Usefulness of photic stimulation in routine clinical electroencephalography. *Neurology* 1960;**10**:777–782.

Jeavons PM, Harding GFA. *Photosensitive Epilepsy. A Review of the Literature and a Study of 460 Patients.* London: Heinemann, 1975.

Patel VM, Maulsby RL. How hyperventilation alters the electroencephalogram: A review of controversial viewpoints emphasizing neurophysiological mechanisms. *J Clin Neurophysiol* 1987;**4**:101–120.

Pratt KL, Mattson RH, Welkers NJ, Williams R. EEG-activation of epileptics following sleep deprivation: a prospective study of 114 cases. *Electroenceph Clin Neurophysiol* 1968; **24**:11–15.

Reilly EL, Peters JF. Relationship of some varieties of electroencephalographic photosensitivity to clinical convulsive disorders. *Neurology* 1973;**23**:1050–1057.

Rowan AJ, Veldhuisen RJ, Nagelkerke ND. Comparative evaluation of sleep deprivation and sedated sleep EEGs as diagnostic aids in epilepsy. *Electroenceph Clin Neurophysiol* 1982; **54**:357–364.

Rowan AJ, Siegel M, Rosenbaum DH. Daytime intensive monitoring: comparison with prolonged intensive and ambulatory monitoring. *Neurology* 1987;**37**:481–484.

Veldhuizen R, Binnie CD, Beinema DJ. The effect of sleep deprivation on the EEG in epilepsy. *Electroenceph Clin Neurophysiol* 1983;**55**:505.

## Normal Variants and Paroxysmal Phenomena of Uncertain Significance

Eeg-Olofsson O. The development of the electroencephalogram in normal children from the age of 1 through 15 years. 14 and 6 positive spike phenomenon. *Neuropaediatrie* 1971; **2**:405–427.

Hugns JR, Cayaffa JJ. Is the "psychomotor variant" "rhythmic mid-temporal discharge" an ictal pattern? *Clin EEG* 1973;**4**:42–49.

Klass DW, Westmoreland BF. Nonepileptogenic epileptiform electroencephalographic activity. *Ann Neurol* 1985;**18**:627–635.

Lipman IJ, Hughes JR. Rhythmic midtemporal discharges. An electroclinical study. *Electroenceph Clin Neurophysiol* 1969;**27**:43–47.

Maulsby RL. EEG patterns of uncertain diagnostic significance. In: DW Klass, DD Daly (eds), *Current Practice of Clinical Electroencephalography.* New York: Raven Press, 1979;411–419.

Miller CR, Westmoreland BF, Klass DW. Subclinical rhythmic EEG discharge of adults (SREDA): Further observations. *Am J EEG Technol* 1985;**25**:217–224.

Pedley TA. EEG patterns that mimic epileptiform discharges but have no association with seizures. In: C Henry (ed.), *Current Clinical Neurophysiology.* Amsterdam: Elsevier, 1981;307–336.

Reiher J, Lebel M. Wicket spikes: Clinical correlates of a previously undescribed EEG pattern. *Can J Neurol Sci* 1977;**4**:39–47.

Thomas JE, Klass DW. Six-per-second spike-and-wave pattern in the electroencephalogram: A reappraisal of its clinical significance. *Neurology* 1968;**18**:587–593.

Westmoreland BF, Klass DW. Midline theta rhythm. *Arch Neurol* 1986;**43**:139–141.

Westmoreland BF, Reiher J, Klass DW. Recording small sharp spikes with depth electroencephalography. *Epilepsia* 1979;**20**:599–606.

Westmoreland BF, Klass DW. Unusual variants of subclinical rhythmic electrographic discharge of adults (SREDA). *Electroenceph Clin Neurophysiol* 1997;**102**:1–4.

White JC, Langston JW, Pedley TA. Benign epileptiform transients of sleep. *Neurology* 1977;**27**:1061–1068.

## Chapter 3: The Abnormal EEG

### Non-epileptiform Abnormal Patterns

Burger L, Rowan AJ, Goldensohn ES. Creutzfeldt-Jakob disease: an electroencephalographic study. *Arch Neurol* 1972;**26**:428–433.

Celesia GG. Pathophysiology of periodic EEG complexes in subacute sclerosing panencephalitis (SSPE). *Electroenceph Clin Neurophysiol* 1973;**35**:293–300.

Chatrian GE, Shaw CM, Leffman H. The significance of periodic lateralized epileptiform discharges in EEG: An electrographic, clinical and pathological study. *Electroenceph Clin Neurophysiol* 1964;**17**:177–193.

Chiofalo N, Fuentes A, Galves C. Serial EEG findings in 27 cases of Creutzfeldt-Jakob disease. *Arch Neurol* 1980;**37**:143–145.

Daly DD, Whelen JL, Bickford RG *et al.* The electroencephalogram in cases of tumors of the posterior fossa and third ventricle. *Electroenceph Clin Neurophysiol* 1953;**5**:203–216.

Daly DD, Markan ON. Focal brain lesions. In: D Daly, T Pedley (eds), *Current Practice of Clinical Electroencephalography*, 2nd edition. New York: Raven Press, 1990;335–370.

Garcia-Morales I, Garcia MT, Galan-Davila L, Gomez-Escalonilla C, Saiz-Diaz R, Martinez-Salio A, de la Pena P, Tejerina JA. Periodic lateralized epileptiform discharges: etiology, clinical aspects, seizures, and evolution in 130 patients. *J Clin Neurophysiol* 2002; **19**:172–177.

Gilmore PC, Brenner RP. Correlation of EEG, computerized tomography, and clinical findings: study of 100 patients with focal delta activity. *Arch Neurol* 1981;**38**:371–372.

Gloor P, Kalaby O, Giard N. The electroencephalogram in diffuse encephalopathies: Electroencephalographic correlates of grey and white matter lesions. *Brain* 1968;**91**:779–802.

Gloor P, Ball G, Schaul N. Brain lesions that produce delta waves in the EEG. *Neurology* 1977;**27**:326–333.

Goldensohn ES. Use of the EEG for evaluation of focal intracranial lesions. In: DW Klass, D Daly (eds), *Current Practice of Clinical Electroencephalography*. New York: Raven Press, 1979;307–342.

Kuroiwa Y, Celesia GG. Clinical significance of periodic EEG patterns. *Arch Neurol* 1980;**37**:15–20.

Lai CW, Gragasin ME. Electroencephalography in herpes simplex encephalitis. *J Clin Neurophysiol* 1988;**5**:87–103.

Levy SR, Chiappa KH, Burke CJ, Young RR. Early evolution and incidence of electroencephalographic abnormalities in Creutzfeldt-Jacob disease. *J Clin Neurophysiol* 1986;**3**:1–21.

Markand ON, Panszi JG. The electroencephalogram in subacute sclerosing panencephalitis (SSPE). *Arch Neurol* 1975;**32**:719–726.

Markand ON. Electroencephalography in diffuse encephalopathies. *J Clin Neurophysiol* 1984;**1**:357–407.

Marshall D, Brey RL, Morse MW. Focal and/or lateralized polymorphic delta activity. *Arch Neurol* 1988;**45**:33–35.

Normand MM, Wszolek ZK, Klass DW. Temporal intermittent rhythmic delta activity in electroencephalograms. *J Clin Neurophysiol* 1995;**12**:280–284.

Pohlmann-Eden B, Hoch DB, Cochius JI, Chiappa KH. Periodic lateralized epileptiform discharges – a critical review. *J Clin Neurophysiol* 1996;**14**:150–153.

Reither J, Rivest J, Grand'Maison F, Leduc CP. Periodic lateralized epileptiform discharges with transitional rhythmic discharges: association with seizures. *Electroenceph Clin Neurophysiol* 1991;**78**:12–17.

Roberts MA, McGeorge AP, Caird FI. Electroencephalography and computerised tomography in vascular and non-vascular dementia in old age. *J Neurol Neurosurg Psychiatr* 1978;**41**:903–906.

Schraeder PI, Singh N. Seizure disorders following periodic lateralized epileptiform discharges. *Epilepsia* 1980;**21**:647–653.

Shaul N, Gloor P, Gotman J. The EEG in deep midline lesions. *Neurology* 1981;**31**:157–167.

Schaul N, Lueders H, Sachdev K. Generalized bilaterally synchronous bursts of slow waves in the EEG. *Arch Neurol* 1981;**38**:690–692.

Sharbrough FW. Nonspecific abnormal EEG patterns. In: E Niedermeyer, F Lopes da Silva (eds), *Electroencephalography: Basic Principles, Clinical Applications and Related Fields.* Baltimore: Urban and Schwarzenberg, 1987;163–182.

Smith JB, Westmoreland BF, Reagan TJ, Sandok BA. A distinctive clinical EEG profile in herpes simplex encephalitis. *Mayo Clin Proc* 1975;**50**:469–474.

Snodgrass SM, Tsuburaya K, Ajmone-Marsan C. Clinical significance of periodic lateralized epileptiform discharges: relationship with status epilepticus. *J Clin Neurophysiol* 1989;**6**:159–172.

Walsh JM, Brenner RP. Periodic lateralized epileptiform discharges: long term outcome in adults. *Epilepsia* 1987;**28**:533–536.

Westmoreland BF, Saunders MG. The EEG in the evaluation of disorders affecting the brain diffusely. In: DW Klass, D Daly (eds), *Current Practice of Clinical Electroencephalography.* New York: Raven Press, 1979;307–342.

Westmoreland BF, Klass DW, Sharbrough FW. Chronic periodic lateralized epileptiform discharges. *Arch Neurol* 1986;**27**:729–733.

## Epileptiform Patterns

Ajmone-Marsan C. Depth electrography and electrocorticography. In: MI Aminoff (ed.), *Electrodiagnosis in Clinical Neurology.* New York: Churchill Livingstone, 1980;167–196.

Blume WT, Lemieux JF. Morphology of spikes in spike-and-wave complexes. *Electroenceph Clin Neurophysiol* 1988;**69**:508–515.

Brazier MAB. Spread of seizure discharges in epilepsy: anatomical and electrophysiological considerations. *Exp Neurol* 1972;**36**:253–272.

Gloor P. Generalized epilepsy with spike-and-wave discharge: A reinterpretation of its electrographic and clinical manifestations. *Epilepsia* 1979;**20**:571–588.

Hrachovy RA, Frost Jr, JD. Infantile spasms. *Cleve Clin J Med* 1989;**56** (Suppl. 1):S10–S16.

Hughs JR. The significance of the interictal spike discharge: A review. *J Clin Neurophysiol* 1989;**6**:207–226.

Kelleway P. The incidence, significance and natural history of spike foci in children. In: CE Henry (ed.). *Current Clinical Neurophysiology.* Amsterdam: Elsevier, 1981;151–175.

Klass DW. Electroencephalographic manifestations of complex partial seizures. In: JK Penry, DD Daly (eds), *Advances in Neurology*, Volume 11. New York: Raven, 1975; 113–140.

Loiseau P, Duche B. Benign childhood epilepsy with centromidtemporal spikes. *Cleve Clin J Med* 1989; **56** (Suppl. 1):S17–S22.

Luders H, Lesser RP, Dinner DS, Morris HH. Benign focal epilepsy of childhood. In: H Lueders, RP Lesser (eds), *Epilepsy: Electroclinical Syndromes.* New York: Springer, 1987;279–302.

Ludwig BI, Ajmone-Marsan, C. Clinical ictal patterns in epileptic patients with occipital electroencephalographic foci. *Neurology* 1975;**25**:462–471.

Niedermeyer E. Abnormal EEG patterns: epileptic and paroxysmal. In: E Niedermeyer, F Lopes da Silva (eds), *Electroencephalography: Basic Principles, Clinical Applications and Related Fields*. Baltimore: Urban and Schwarzenberg, 1993;217–240.

Panayiotopoulos CP. Benign childhood epilepsy with occipital paroxysms: A 15-year prospective study. *Ann Neurol* 1989;**26**:51–56.

Pedley TA, Tharp BR, Herman K. Clinical and electroencephalographic characteristics of midline parasagittal foci. *Ann Neurol* 1981;**9**:142–149.

Pourmand RA, Markand ON, Thomas C. Midline spike discharges: Clinical and EEG correlations. *Clin EEG* 1984;**15**:232–237.

Schwartzkroin PA, Wyler AR. Mechanisms underlying epileptiform burst discharge. *Ann Neurol* 1980;**7**:95–107.

Walczak TS, Jayakar P. Interictal EEG. In: J Engel Jr, TA Pedley (eds), *Epilepsy. A Comprehensive Textbook*, Volume 1. Philadelphia: Lippincott, 1998;831–848.

Westmoreland BF. The electroencephalogram in patients with epilepsy. In: MJ Aminoff (ed.), *Electrodiagnosis in Clinical Neurology*. Philadelphia: WB Saunders, 1985;599–614.

Westmoreland BF, Gomez MR. Infantile Spasms (West Syndrome). In: H Lueders, RP Lesser (eds), *Epilepsy: Electroclinical Syndromes*. New York: Springer, 1987;49–72.

Zivin L, Ajmone Marsan C. Incidence and prognostic significance of "epileptiform activity" in the EEG of non-epileptic patients. *Brain* 1968;**91**:751–778.

## Chapter 4: The EEG and Epilepsy

### Eight Important Epilepsy Syndromes

Aicardi J, Levy Gomes A. Clinical and electroencephalographic symptomatology of the "genuine" Lennox–Gastaut syndrome and its differentiation from other forms of epilepsy of early childhood. *Epilepsy Res Suppl* 1992;**6**:185–193.

Andermann F, Salanova V, Olivier A, Rasmussen T. Occipital lobe epilepsy in children – electroclinical manifestations, surgical indications and treatment. In: F Andermann, A Beaumanoir, L Mira, J Roger, CA Tassinari (eds), *Occipital Seizures and Epilepsies in Children*. London, England: John Libby & Co, 1993;213–220.

Andermann F, Zifkin B. The benign occipital epilepsies of childhood: an overview of the idiopathic syndromes and of the relationship to migraine. *Epilepsia* 1998;**39** (suppl. 4): S9–S23.

Beaussart M. Benign epilepsy of children with Rolandic (centro-temporal) paroxysmal foci. A clinical entity. Study of 221 cases. *Epilepsia* 1972;**13**:795–811.

Beaumanoir A, Ballist T, Varfis G, *et al*. Benign epilepsy of childhood with Rolandic spikes. *Epilepsia* 1974;**15**:301–315.

Blume WT. Lennox–Gastaut Syndrome. In: H Lueders, RP Lesser RP (eds), *Epilepsy: Electroclinical Syndromes*. New York: Springer, 1987;73–92.

Browne TR, Penry JK, Porter RJ, Dreifuss FE. Responsiveness before, during and after spike-wave paroxysms. *Neurology* 1974;**24**:659–665.

Delgado-Escueta AV, Enrile-Bacsal F. Juvenile myoclonic epilepsy of Janz. *Neurology* 1984;**34**:285–294.

Delgado-Escueta AV, Serratosa JM, Liu A, Weissbecker K, *et al*. Progress in mapping human epilepsy genes. *Epilepsia* 1994;**35** (suppl. 1):29–40.

Dieter J. Juvenile myoclonic epilepsy. *Cleve Clin J Med* 1989; **56** (suppl. 1):S23–S33.

Fitzgerald LF, Stone JI, Highes JR, Melyn MA, Lansky LL. The Lennox–Gastaut syndrome: electroencephalographic characteristics, clinical correlates, and follow-up studies. *Clin Electroencephalogr* 1992;**23**:180–189.

Gastaut H. A new type of epilepsy: benign partial epilepsy of childhood with occipital spike-waves. *Clin EEG* 1982;**13**:13–22.

Gomez MR, Westmoreland BF. Absence seizures. In: H Lueders, RP Lesser (eds), *Epilepsy: Electroclinical Syndromes*. London: Springer, 1987;105–129.

Hrachovy RA, Frost Jr, JD. Infantile spasms. *Cleve Clin J Med* 1989;**56** (suppl. 1): S10–S16.

Lee SI. Electroencephalography in infantile and childhood epilepsy. In: FE Dreifuss (ed.), *Pediatric Epileptology*. Boston: Hohn Wright, 1983;33–64.

Loiseau P. Childhood absence epilepsy. In: J Roger, C Dravet, M Bureau (eds), *Epileptic Syndromes in Infancy, Childhood and Adolescence*. London: John Libbey Eurotext, 1985;106–120.

Loiseau P, Duche B. Benign childhood epilepsy with centromidtemporal spikes. *Cleve Clin J Med* 1989;**56** (suppl. 1):S17–S22.

Lueders H, Lesser RP, Dinner DS, Morris HH. Generalized epilepsies: A review. *Cleve Clin Q* 1984;**51**:205–226.

Martinovic Z. Clinical correlations of electroencephalographic occipital epileptiform paroxysms in children. *Seizure* 2001;**10**:379–381.

Panayiotopoulos CP. Benign childhood epilepsy with occipital paroxysms: a 15-year prospective study. *Ann Neurol* 1989;**26**:51–56.

Panayiotopoulos CP. Visual phenomena and headache in occipital epilepsy: a review, a systematic study and differentiation from migraine. *Epileptic Disord* 1999;**1**:205–216.

Penry JK, Porter RJ, Dreifuss FE. Simultaneous recording of absence seizures with video tape and electroencephalography. A study of 374 seizures in 48 patients. *Brain* 1975; **98**:427–440.

Talwar D, Rask CA, Torres F. Clinical manifestations in children with occipital spike-wave paroxysms. *Epilepsia* 1992;**33**:667–674.

Weinmann HM. Lennox–Gastaut syndrome and its relationship to infantile spasms (West syndrome). In: E Niedermeyer, R Degen (eds), *The Lennox–Gastaut Syndrome*. New York, NY: Alan R Liss Inc, 1988;301–316.

Westmoreland BF, Gomez MR. Infantile spasms (West syndrome). In: H Lueders, RP Lesser (eds), *Epilepsy: Electroclinical syndromes*. New York: Springer, 1987;49–72.

Wolf P. Epileptic seizures and syndromes: terms and concepts. In: P Wolf (ed.), *Epileptic Seizures and Syndromes*. London: John Libby, 1994;3–7.

## The Value of the EEG in Epilepsy Prognosis

Callaghan N, Garrett A, Googin T. Withdrawal of anticonvulsant drugs in patients free of seizures for two years. *N Engl J Med* 1988;**318**:942–946.

Juul-Jensen P. Frequency of seizure recurrence after discontinuance of anticonvulsant medication in patients with epileptic seizures. *Epilepsia* 1964;**5**:352–363.

Medical Research Council Antiepileptic Drug Withdrawal Study Group. Randomized study of antiepileptic drug withdrawal in patients in remission. *Lancet* 1991;**337**:1175–1180.

Overweg J, Binnie CD, Oosting J, Rowan AJ. Clinical and EEG prediction of seizure recurrence following antiepileptic drug withdrawal. *Epilepsy Res* 1987;**1**:272–283.

Shafer SQ, Hauser WA, Annegers JF, Klass DW. EEG and other early predictors of epilepsy remission: a community study. *Epilepsia* 1988;**29**:580–600.

Shinnar S, Vining EPG, Mellits ED, D'Sousa BJ *et al*. Discontinuing antiepileptic medication in children with epilepsy after two years without seizures. *N Engl J Med* 1985; **313**:976–980.

## Epilepsy Monitoring

Adams DJ, Lueders H. Hyperventilation and 6-hour EEG recording in evaluation of absence seizures. *Neurology* 1981;**31**:1175–1177.

Binnie CD, Rowan AJ. Prolonged EEG and video monitoring in epilepsy. An evaluation study. *Neurology* 1981;**31**:298–303.

Gumnit RJ (ed.), *Intensive Diagnostic Monitoring. Advances in Neurology*, Volume 46. New York: Raven Press, 1987.

Porter RJ, Sato S, Long RL. Video recording. *Electroenceph Clin Neurophysiol* 1985;**37** (suppl.):73–82.

Porter RJ, Sato S. Prolonged EEG and video monitoring in the diagnosis of seizure disorders. In: E Niedermeyer, FH Lopes da Silva (eds), *Electroencephalography: Basic Principles, Clinical Applications and Related Fields*. Baltimore: Urban and Schwarzenberg, 1987; 634–644.

## The EEG in Non-epileptic Seizures of Psychogenic Origin

Gates JR, Ramani V, Whalen S, Loewenson R. Ictal characteristics of pseudoseizures. *Arch Neurol* 1985;**42**:1183–1187.

Gumnit RJ, Gates JF. Psychogenic seizures. *Epilepsia* 1986;**27**:5124–5129.

King DW, Gallagher BB, Murvin AJ, Smith DB *et al*. Pseudoseizures: diagnosis, evaluation. *Neurology* 1982;**32**:18–23.

## Status Epilepticus

Aminoff MJ, Simon RP. Status epilepticus. Causes, clinical features and consequences in 98 patients. *Am J Med* 1980;**69**:657–666.

Boggs JG, Towne AR, Smith J, Pellock JM, DeLorenzo RJ. Frequency of potentially ictal patterns in comatose ICU patients. *Epilepsia* 1994;**35**:135.

Brenner RP. Is it status? *Epilepsia* 2002;**43** (suppl. 3):103–113.

Casino GD. Nonconvulsive status epilepticus in adults and children. *Epilepsia* 1993;**34**:781–784.

Dodrill CB, Wilensky AJ. Intellectual impairment as an outcome of status epilepticus. *Neurology* 1990;**40**:23–27.

Drislane FW Evidence against permanent neurologic damage from nonconvulsive status epilepticus. *J Clin Neurophysiol* 1999;**16**:323–331.

Granner MA, Lee SI. Nonconvulsive status epilepticus: EEG analysis in a large series. *Epilepsia* 1994;**35**:42–47.

Kaplan PW. Assessing the outcomes in patients with nonconvulsive status epilepticus: nonconvulsive status epilepticus in underdiagnosed, potentially over treated, and confounded by comorbidity. *J Clin Neurophysiol* 1999;**16**:341–352.

Kaplan PW. Prognosis in nonconvulsive status epilepticus. *Epileptic Disord* 2000;**2**:185–193.

Mayer SA, Claassen J, Lokin J, Mendelsohn F, Dennis LJ, Fitzsimmons BF. Refractory status epilepticus: frequency, risk factors, and impact on outcome. *Arch Neurol* 2002;**59**:205–210.

Porter RJ, Penry JK. Petit mal status. *Adv Neurol* 1983;**34**:61–67.

Privitera M, Hoffman M, Moore JL, Jester D. EEG detection of nontonic-clonic status epilepticus in patients with altered consciousness. *Epilepsy Res* 1994;**18**:155–166.

Rowan AJ, Scott DF. Major status epilepticus. *Acta Neurol Scand* 1970;**446**:573–584.

Towne AR, Waterhouse EJ, Boggs JG, Garnett LK, Brown AJ, Smith JR Jr, DeLorenzo RJ. Prevalence of nonconvulsive status epilepticus in comatose patients. *Neurology* 2000;**54**:340–345.

Treiman DM, Walton NY, Kendrick C. A progressive sequence of electroencephalographic changes during generalized convulsive status epilepticus. *Epilepsy Res* 1990;**5**:49–60.

Treiman DM, Meyers PD, Walton NY, Collins JF, Rowan AJ, Handforth A, Faught E, Calabrese VP, Uthman BM, Ramsay RE, Mamdani MB, Yagnik P, Jones JC, Berry E, Boggs JG, Kanner AM. Treatment of generalized convulsive status epilepticus: a randomized double-blind comparison of four intravenous regimens. *N Engl J Med* 1998;**339**:792–798.

Waterhouse EJ, DeLorenzo RJ. Status epilepticus in older patients: epidemiology and treatment options. *Drugs Aging* 2001;**18**:133–142.

## Chapter 5: The EEG in Other Neurological and Medical Conditions

### The Dementias

Burger L, Rowan AJ, Goldensohn ES. Creutzfeldt-Jakob disease: an electroencephalographic study. *Arch Neurol* 1972;**26**:428–433.

Chiofalo NN, Fuentes A, Galve C. Serial EEG findings in 27 cases of Creutzfeldt-Jakob disease. *Arch Neurol* 1980;**37**:143–145.

Gloor P, Kalaby O, Giard N. The electroencephalogram in diffuse encephalopathies: electroencephalographic correlates of grey and white matter lesions. *Brain* 1968;**91**: 779–802.

Harner RN. EEG evaluation of the patient with dementia. In: DF Benson, D Blumer (eds), *Psychiatric Aspects of Neurological Disease*. New York: Grune and Stratton, 1975: 63–82.

Levy SR, Chiappa KH, Burke CJ, Young RR. Early evolution and incidence of electroencephalographic abnormalities in Creutzfeldt-Jakob disease. *J Clin Neurophysiol* 1986; **3**:1–21.

Markand ON. Electroencephalography in diffuse encephalopathies. *J Clin Neurophysiol* 1984; **1**:357–407.

Roberts MA, McGeorge AP, Caird FI. Electroencephalography and computerised tomography in vascular and non-vascular dementia in old age. *J Neurol Neurosurg Psychiatr* 1978; **41**:903–906.

Westmoreland BF, Saunders MG. The EEG in the evaluation of disorders affecting the brain diffusely. In: DW Klass, D Daly (eds), *Current Practice of Clinical Electroencephalography*. New York: Raven Press, 1979;307–342.

### Stroke

Goldensohn ES. Use of the EEG for evaluation of focal intracranial lesions. In: DW Klass, D Daly (eds), *Current Practice of Clinical Electroencephalography*, New York: Raven Press, 1979;307–342.

MacDonnell RAL, Donnan GA, Bladin PF, Berkovic SF, Wriedt CHR. The electroencephalogram and acute ischemic stroke. Distinguishing cortical from lacunar infarction. *Arch Neurol* 1988;**45**:520–524.

Petty GW, Labar DR, Fisch BJ, Pedley TA, Mohr JP, Khandiji A. EEG in lacunar strokes. *Ann Neurol* 1988;**24**:129A.

Van der Drift JHA, Kok NKD. Section II. The EEG in cerebrovascular disorders in relation to pathology. In: A Remond (ed.), *Handbook of Electroencephalography and Clinical Neurophysiology*, Volume 14A. Amsterdam: Elsevier, 1975;12–64.

## Subdural Hematoma

Bickford RG, Klass DW. EEG changes with acute and chronic head injury. In: EF Caveness, E Walker (eds), *Head Injury Conference Proceedings*. Philadelphia: Lippincott, 1966.

## Metabolic Disorders

Bickford RG, Butts HR. Hepatic coma: the electroencephalographic pattern. *J Clin Invest* 1955;**34**:790–799.

Cadilhac J. EEG in thyroid dysfunction. In: GH Glaser (ed.), *Handbook of Electroencephalography and Clinical Neurophysiology*. Amsterdam: Elsevier, 1976:**15C**;70–76.

Foley JM, Watson CW, Adams RD. Significance of the electroencephalographic changes in hepatic coma. *Trans Am Neurol Assoc* 1950;**75**:161–165.

Harner RN, Katz RI. Section IV. Electroencephalography in metabolic coma. In: A Remond (ed.), *Handbook of Electroencephalography and Clinical Neurophysiology*, Volume 12. Amsterdam: Elsevier, 1975:47–62.

Mahurkar SD, Dhar SK, Salta R, Meyers L, Smith EC, Dunea G. Dialysis dementia. *Lancet* 1973;**1**:1412–1415.

Markand ON. Electroencephalography in diffuse encephalopathies. *J Clin Neurophysiol* 1984;**1**:357–407.

Silverman D. Some observations on the EEG in hepatic coma. *Electroenceph Clin Neurophysiol* 1962;**14**:53–59.

Swash, M, Rowan AJ. The electroencephalographic criteria of hypocalcemia and hypercalcemia. *Arch Neurol* 1972;**26**:218–228.

Westmoreland BF, Saunders MG. The EEG in the evaluation of disorders affecting the brain diffusely. In: DW Klass, D Daly (eds), *Current Practice of Clinical Electroencephalography*. New York: Raven Press, 1979;307–342.

## Coma

Austin EJ, Wilkus R, Longstreath WT. Etiology and prognosis of alpha coma. *Neurology* 1988;**38**:773–777.

Brenner RP. The electroencephalogram in altered states of consciousness. In: MJ Aminoff (ed.), *Electrodiagnosis, Neurologic Clinics*. Philadelphia, Saunders, 1985;615–629.

Britt Jr. CW, Raso E, Gerson P. Spindle coma, secondary to primary traumatic midbrain hemorrhage. *Electroenceph Clin Neurophysiol* 1980;**49**:406–408.

Harner RN, Katz RI. Section IV. Electroencephalography in metabolic coma. In: A Remond (ed.), *Handbook of Electroencephalography and Clinical Neurophysiology*, Volume 12. Amsterdam: Elsevier, 1975;47–62.

Sorenson K, Thomassen A, Wernberg M. Prognostic significance of alpha frequency EEG rhythm in coma after cardiac arrest. *J Neurol Neurosurg Psychiatr* 1978;**41**:840–842.

Westmoreland BF, Klass DW, Sharbrough FW, Reagan TJ. Alpha-coma. Electroencephalographic, clinical, pathologic, and etiologic correlations. *Arch Neurol* 1975;**32**: 713–718.

Zaret BS. Prognostic and neurophysiological implications of concurrent burst suppression and alpha patterns in the EEG of post-anoxic coma. *Electroenceph Clin Neurophysiol* 1985;**61**:199–209.

## Chapter 6: Tips on Reading and Reporting the EEG

American EEG Society Guidelines in Electroencephalography, Evoked Potentials and Polysomnography. Guideline Eight: Guidelines for writing EEG reports. *J Clin Neurophysiol* 1994;**11**:37–39.

Kellaway P. An orderly approach to visual analysis: parameters of the normal EEG in adults and children. In: DW Klass, DD Daly (eds), *Current Practice of Clinical Electroencephalography*. New York: Raven Press, 1979;69–147.

Schneider J. Section IV. The EEG report. In: A Remond (ed.), *Handbook of Electroencephalography and Clinical Neurophysiology*, Volume II A. Amsterdam: Elsevier, 1977;97–109.

# APPENDIX

## The Influence of Pharmacological Agents on the EEG/Role of the EEG in Determining Anti-epileptic Drug Therapy

Brazier MAB. Studies of electrical activity of the brain in relation to anesthesia. In: Abramson HA (ed.), *Conference on Neuropharmacology*. New York: Josiah Macy Jr Foundation, 1955;107–144.

Denny-Brown DE, Swan RL, Foley IM. Respiratory and electrical signs in barbiturate intoxications. *Trans Am Neurol Assoc* 1947;**77**:77.

Eriksson AS, Knutsson E, Nergardh A. The effect of lamotrigine on epileptiform discharges in young patients with drug-resistant epilepsy. *Epilepsia* 2001;**42**:230–236.

Fink M. EEG and human psychopharmacology. *Annu Rev Pharmacol* 1968;**9**:241–258.

Frost JD Jr, Hrachovy RA, Glaze DG, Rettig GM. Alpha rhythm slowing during initiation of carbamazepine therapy: implications for future cognitive performance. *J Clin Neurophysiol* 1995;**12**:57–63.

Gibbs FA, Gibbs EL, Lennox WG. Effect on the electroencephalogram of certain drugs which influence nervous activity. *Arch Intern Med* 1937;**60**:154–166.

Haider J, Matthew H, Oswald J. Electroencephalographic changes in acute drug poisoning. *Electroenceph Clin Neurophysiol* 1971;**30**:23–31.

Harvey SC. Hypnotics and sedatives. The barbiturates. In: Goodman LS, Gilman A (eds), *The Pharmacological Basis of Therapeutics*. New York: Macmillan, 1975;102–123.

Herkes GK, Lagerlund TD, Sharbrough FW, Eadie MJ. Effects of antiepileptic drug treatment on the background frequency of EEGs in epileptic patients. *J Clin Neurophysiol* 1993;**10**:210–216.

Hollister LE, Barthel CA. Changes in the electroencephalogram during chronic administration of the tranquilizing drugs. *Electroenceph Clin Neurophysiol* 1959;**11**:792–795.

Kalviainen R, Aikia M, Mervaala E, Saukkonen AM, Pitkanen A, Riekkinen PJ Sr. Long-term cognitive and EEG effects of tiagabine in drug-resistant partial epilepsy. *Epilepsy Res* 1996;**25**:291–297.

Kochen S, Giagante B, Oddo S. Spike-wave complexes and seizure exacerbation caused by carbamazepine. *Eur J Neurol* 2002;**9**:41–47.

Kugler J, Lorenzi E, Spatz R, Zimmerman H. Drug-induced paroxysmal EEG activities. *Pharmacopsychiatry* 1979;**12**:165–172.

Kurtz D. The EEG in acute and chronic drug intoxications. In: Glaser GH (ed.), *Metabolic and Toxic Diseases/Handbook of Electroencephalography and Clinical Neurophysiology*, Volume 15. Amsterdam: Elsevier, 1976;88–104.

Marciani MG, Gigli GL, Stefanini F, Sabbadini M, Stefani N, Maschio MC, Orlandi L, Bernardi G. Effect of carbamazepine on EEG background activity and on interictal epileptiform abnormalities in focal epilepsy. *Int J Neurosci* 1993;**70**:107–116.

Marciani MG, Stanzione P, Maschio M, Spanedda F, Bassetti MA, Mattia D, Bernardi G. EEG changes induced by vigabatrin monotherapy in focal epilepsy. *Acta Neurol Scand* 1997;**95**:115–120.

Marciani MG, Stanzione P, Mattia D, Spanedda F, Bassetti MA, Maschio M, Bernardi G. Lamotrigine add-on therapy in focal epilepsy: electroencephalographic and neuropsychological evaluation. *Clin Neuropharmacol* 1998;**21**:41–47.

Mecarelli O, Piacenti A, Pulitano P, Vicenzini E, Rizzo C, Rinalduzzi S, de Feo MR, Accornero N. Clinical and electroencephalographic effects of topiramate in patients with epilepsy and healthy volunteers. *Clin Neuropharmacol* 2001;**24**:284–289.

Talwar D, Arora MS, Sher PK. EEG changes and seizure exacerbation in young children treated with carbamazepine. *Epilepsia* 1994;**35**:1154–1159.

Toman JEP, Davis JP. The effects of drugs upon the electrical activity of the brain. *J Pharmacol Exp Ther* 1949;**97**:425–492.

Van Sweden B, Dumon-Radermecker M. The EEG in chronic psychotropic drug intoxications. *Clin Electroenceph* 1982;**13**:206–215.

## Guidelines for Treatment of Generalized Convulsive Status Epilepticus (GCSE)

Claassen J, Hirsch LJ, Emerson RG, Mayer SA. Treatment of refractory status epilepticus with pentobarbital, propofol, or midazolam: a systematic review. *Epilepsia* 2002;**43**: 146–153.

DeGiorgio CM, Altman K, Hamilton-Byrd E, Rabinowicz AL. Lidocaine in refractory status epilepticus: confirmation of efficacy with continuous EEG monitoring. *Epilepsia* 1992;**33**: 913–916.

Dodson WE, DeLorenzo RJ, Pedley TA, Shinnar S, Treiman DM, Wannamaker BB. The treatment of convulsive status epilepticus: recommendations of the Epilepsy Foundation of America's Working Group on Status Epilepticus. *JAMA* 1993;**270**: 854–859.

Kumar A, Bleck TP. Intravenous midazolam for the treatment of refractory status epilepticus. *Crit Care Med* 1992;**20**:483–488.

Labar DR, Ali A, Root J. High-dose intravenous lorazepam for the treatment of refractory status epilepticus. *Neurology* 1994;**44**:1400–1403.

Parent JM, Lowenstein DH. Treatment of refractory generalized status epilepticus with continuous infusion of midazolam. *Neurology* 1994;**44**:1837–1840.

Pitt-Miller PL, Elcock BJ, Maharaj M. The management of status epilepticus with a continuous propofol infusion. *Anesth Analg* 1994;**78**:1193–1194.

Treiman DM, Meyers PD, Walton NY, Collins JF, Rowan AJ, Handforth A, Faught E, Calabrese VP, Uthman BM, Ramsay RE, Mamdani MB, Yagnik P, Jones JC, Berry E, Boggs JG, Kanner AM. Treatment of generalized convulsive status epilepticus: a randomized double-blind comparison of four intravenous regimens. *N Engl J Med* 1998;**339**:792–798.

Yaffe K, Lowenstein DH. Prognostic factors of pentobarbital therapy for refractory generalized status epilepticus. *Neurology* 1993;**43**:895–900.

## Guidelines for Treatment of Non-convulsive Status Epilepticus (NCSE)

Begemann M, Rowan AJ, Tuhrim S. Treatment of refractory complex-partial status epilepticus with propofol: case report. *Epilepsia* 2000;**41**:105–109.

Claassen J, Hirsch LJ, Emerson RG, Bates JE, Thompson TB, Mayer SA. Continuous EEG monitoring and midazolam infusion for refractory nonconvulsive status epilepticus. *Neurology* 2001;**57**:1036–1042.

DeLorenzo RJ, Waterhouse EJ, Towne AR, Boggs JG, Ko D, DeLorenzo GA, Brown A, Garnett L. Persistent nonconvulsive status epilepticus after the control of convulsive status epilepticus. *Epilepsia* 1998;**39**:833–840.

Kaplan PW. Do some types of nonconvulsive status epilepticus cause little permanent neurologic sequelae (or: "the cure may be worse than the disease")? *Neurophysiol Clin* 2000;**30**:377–382.

Lee SI. Nonconvulsive status epilepticus. Ictal confusion in later life. *Arch Neurol* 1985;**42**:778–781.

Litt B, Wityk RJ, Hertz SH, Mullen PD, Weiss H, Ryan DD, Henry TR. Nonconvulsive status epilepticus in the critically ill elderly. *Epilepsia* 1998;**39**:1194–1202.

Walker MC. Diagnosis and treatment of nonconvulsive status epilepticus. *CNS Drugs* 2001;**15**:931–939.

Waterhouse EJ, DeLorenzo RJ. Status epilepticus in older patients: epidemiology and treatment options. *Drug Aging* 2001;**18**:133–142.

## Cerebral Death Recording

American Electroencephalographic Society. Guideline three: minimal technical standards for EEG recording in suspected cerebral death. *J Clin Neurophysiol* 1994;**11**:10–13.

Brenner RP, Schwartzman R, Richey E. Prognostic significance of episodic low amplitude or relatively isoelectric EEG patterns. *Dis Nerv Syst* 1975;**36**:582.

Chatrian GE. Electrophysiologic evaluation of brain death: a critical appraisal. In: MJ Aminoff (ed.), *Electrodiagnosis in Clinical Neurology*. New York: Churchill-Livingstone, 1986;669–736.

Jorgensen EO. Requirements for recording the EEG at high sensitivity in suspected brain death. *Electroenceph Clin Neurophysiol* 1974;**36**:65–69.

Wijdicks, EFM. The diagnosis of brain death. *N Engl J Med* 2001:**344**;1215–1221.

# MINI-ATLAS

# EEGs

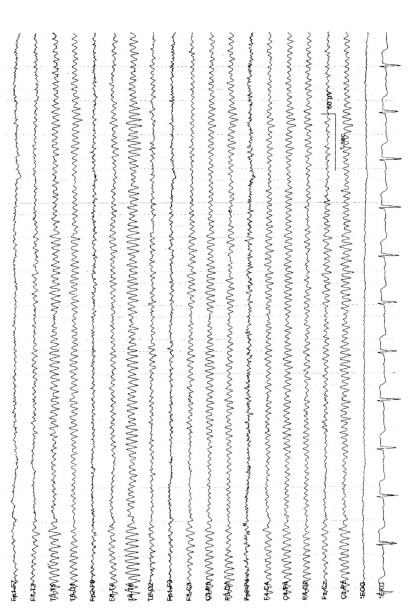

**A-1** Normal adult. This is a 55-year-old man who is awake with eyes closed. There is a well-developed alpha rhythm at 10 Hz, prominent in the posterior head regions. The sinusoidal waves constitute the major and nearly only finding in this record. Little if any beta activity is present.

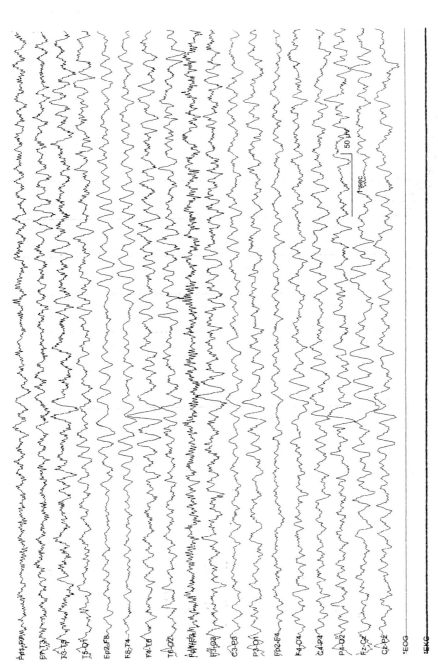

**A-2** Normal 7-month-old. This healthy 7-month-old baby boy has a well-organized background rhythm of about 5 Hz. The rhythmic waves are best seen in the temporal regions and are widely distributed. A few slower frequencies are admixed with the theta, and there is a small amount of beta activity. There is low-voltage muscle artifact in the left frontotemporal region.

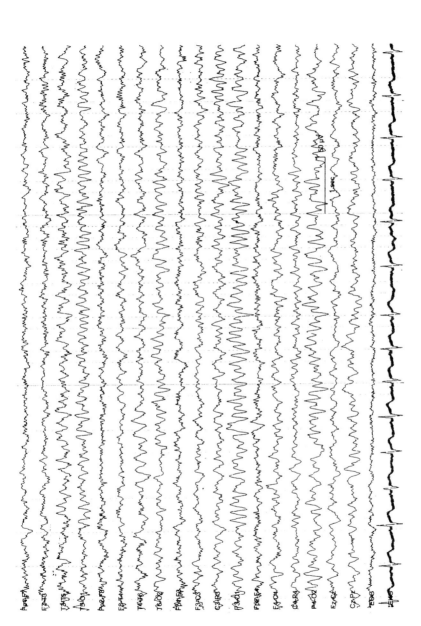

**A-3** Normal 4-year-old. This is a healthy 4-year-old boy with a history of a single febrile convulsion. The background contains a prominent rhythmic frequency at about 7 Hz, well seen in Channels 4, 8, 12, and 16. This is the posterior dominant rhythm. Note the admixed slower frequencies, normal for this age. A small amount of diffuse beta activity is present.

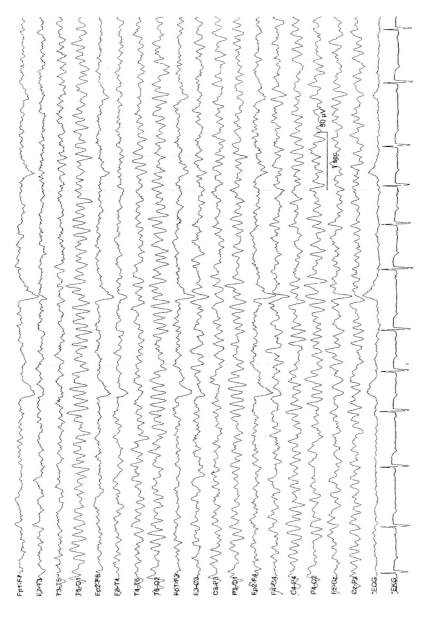

**A-4** Normal 5-year-old. This healthy 5-year-old boy has a very well-organized posterior dominant rhythm of 7 Hz. Note rare admixed slower frequencies along with some more diffuse irregular theta waves. Eye blink artifact is evident in the frontal leads.

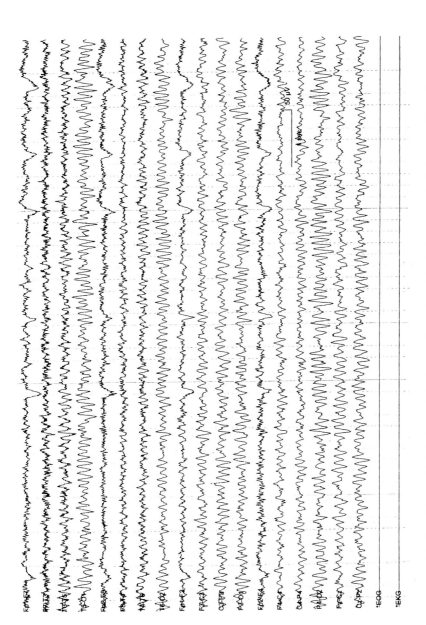

A-5  Normal 8-year-old. This 8-year-old boy has a well-organized alpha rhythm at 9.5 Hz, nicely seen in Channels 4, 8, 12, and 16. Note a small amount of intermingled slower frequencies, fewer than in the previous record. Eye blink artifact is present in the frontal regions (Channels 1, 5, 9, and 13), and a low-voltage muscle artifact is evident in the fronto-temporal derivations.

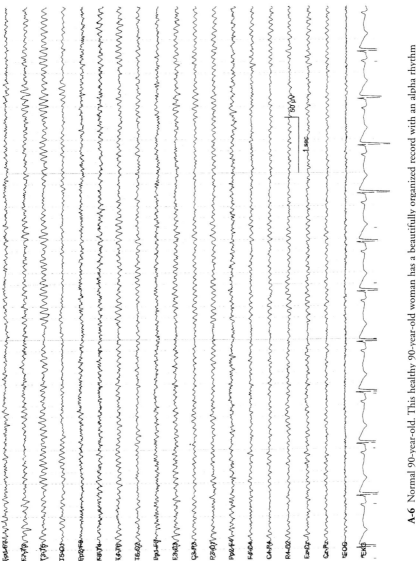

**A-6** Normal 90-year-old. This healthy 90-year-old woman has a beautifully organized record with an alpha rhythm of 9.5 to 10 Hz. A small amount of beta activity is present in the frontal regions. This demonstrates that the EEG may remain normal throughout life.

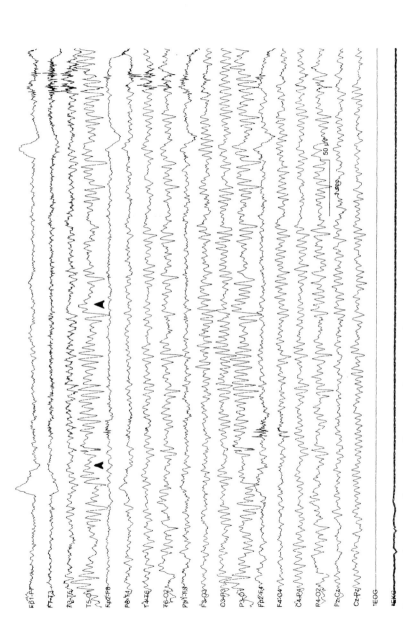

**A-7**  Posterior slow waves of youth. This record, obtained from an adolescent, shows nicely organized alpha activity at 9 Hz, of higher amplitude on the left side. There are frequent sharply contoured delta waves that underlie the alpha, also more prominent on the left. "Youth waves" are common between the ages of 8 to 15 years and may be prominent and frequently recurring. They attenuate with eye-opening, as does the alpha, and should not be interpreted as focal slowing or of paroxysmal significance.

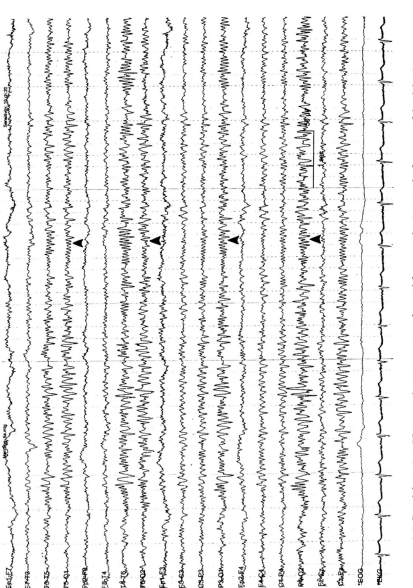

**A-8** Fast alpha variant. This normal variant consists of a rapid frequency that is twice the frequency of the alpha. In this case the variant is prominent in the posterior quadrants at a frequency of 20 Hz. Note the alpha in the same location at 10 Hz. The variant may alternate with the alpha or may predominate with only a small amount of alpha. It has the same general characteristics as the alpha, for example attenuation with eye opening.

A-9 Slow alpha variant. This normal variant is characterized by rhythmic waves that are half the frequency of the alpha. As with fast alpha variant, it may alternate with the alpha or may predominate with little alpha representation. In this example the alpha frequency is 9 Hz, and the variant appears at 4.5 Hz. Suspect a slow alpha variant if there are "notches" on top of the slow rhythmic waves, as is the case here.

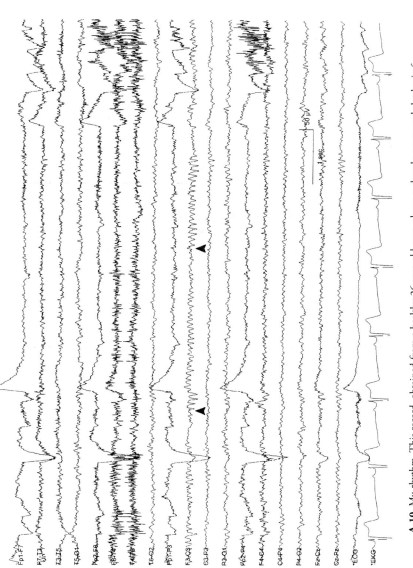

**A-10** Mu rhythm. This record, obtained from a healthy 26-year-old man, shows a sharply contoured rhythmic frequency at 11 Hz in the left centro-parietal region. Mu rhythm consists of arch-shaped waves at a frequency of 7 to 11 Hz, usually maximal over the central regions. Runs of mu are intermittent and may occur independently over the two hemispheres, or may be unilateral. Movement of the contralateral upper extremity (such as making a fist), or even thinking of such movement, attenuates the rhythm.

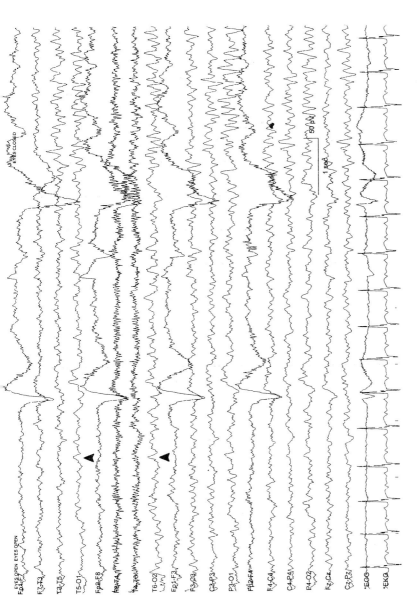

**A-11** Lambda waves. Lambda waves are sharp transients of positive polarity, recorded in the occipital regions. They are generated in the waking state when the subject scans the environment, for example a picture or something else of interest. This example, obtained in a normal 4-year-old boy, demonstrates repetitive lambda waves, best seen in Channels 4 and 8. Note that the subject's eyes are open. An eye blink artifact appears in the 4th second. When he closes his eyes, a somewhat irregular posterior dominant rhythm at 7 to 8 Hz is established.

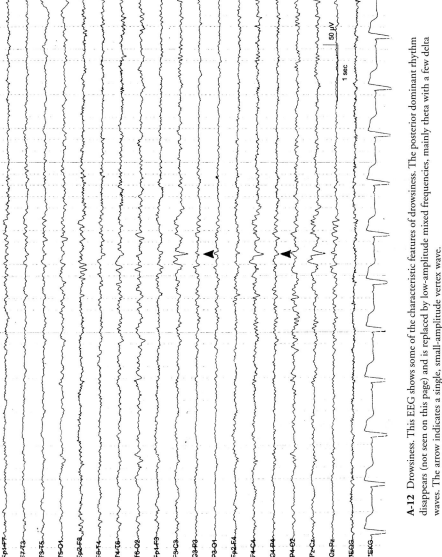

**A-12** Drowsiness. This EEG shows some of the characteristic features of drowsiness. The posterior dominant rhythm disappears (not seen on this page) and is replaced by low-amplitude mixed frequencies, mainly theta with a few delta waves. The arrow indicates a single, small-amplitude vertex wave.

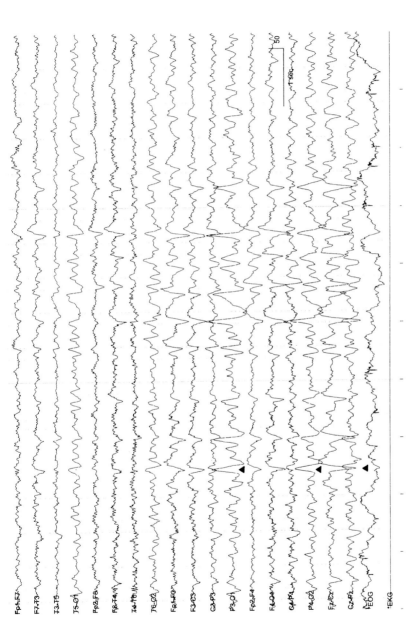

**A-13** Vertex sharp waves (V waves). Vertex sharp waves are normal elements of Stage II sleep but may first appear in drowsiness. They are bilaterally synchronous with maximum focality at the vertex, or sometimes slightly posteriorly. They may appear in isolation or in brief runs, as in this recording. Note the typical morphology, high-amplitude, bilateral synchrony, and phase reversals between the central and parietal electrodes.

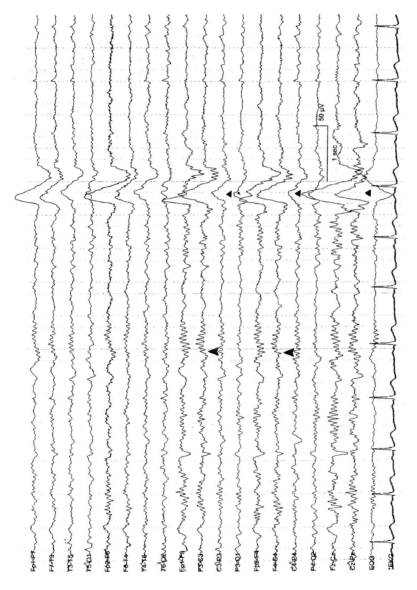

**A-14** Stage II sleep. Stage II sleep is characterized principally by well-developed sleep spindles. Spindles are defined as rhythmic waves at 12 to 14 (± 2) Hz and are maximal over the central regions. K-complexes are high-voltage uni- or biphasic delta waves with a distribution similar to vertex sharp waves. They often, but not invariably, are accompanied by a trailing sleep spindle, as in this case. Note the large arrow indicating the spindle and the small arrow under the K-complex.

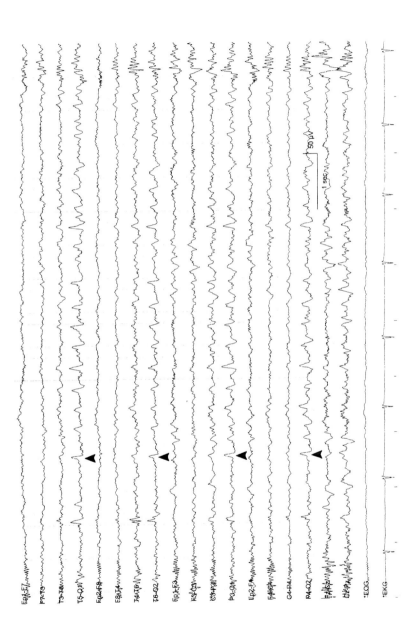

**A-15** POSTS. This EEG demonstrates positive occipital sharp transients of sleep (POSTS) in a run that is quite rhythmic. They appear during Stage II sleep and consist of triangular waves of positive polarity in the occipital regions. POSTS may be synchronous or independent and sometimes are of quite high-voltage with a sharp configuration. It is important that POSTS not be confused with epileptiform sharp waves.

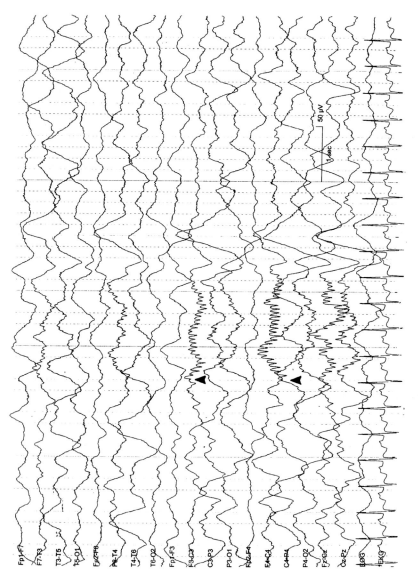

**A-16** Normal sleep in a 5-month-old. This example, obtained in a normal 5-month-old infant, is characterized by high-amplitude delta waves, diffusely distributed. In the central regions note the well-developed sleep spindle at 14 to 15 Hz (indicated by the arrow).

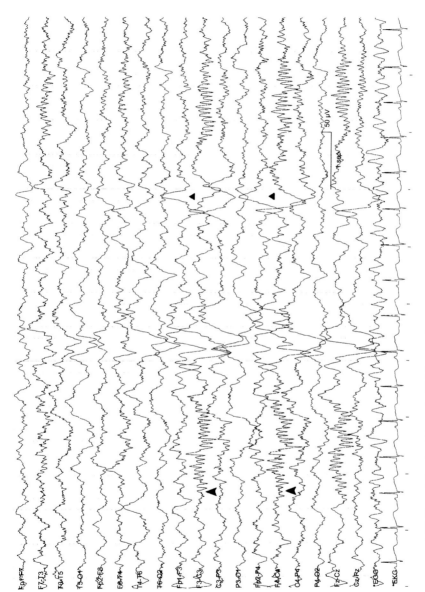

A-17 Normal sleep in a 20-month-old. This recording from a normal 20-month-boy shows a background consisting of an admixture of theta and delta activity. Nicely developed sleep spindles at 14 Hz are evident (large arrow), as are K-complexes (small arrow).

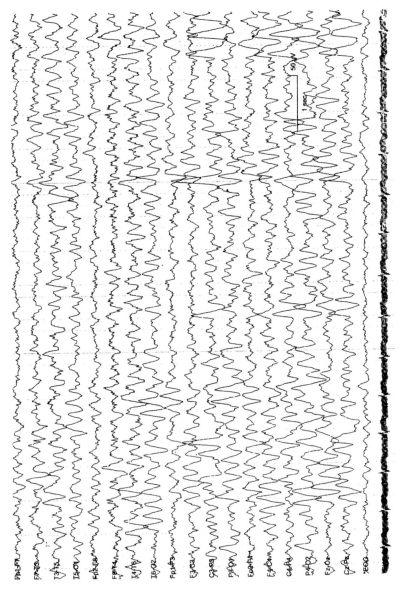

**A-18** Hypnagogic hypersynchrony. This is a normal 2-year-old boy who is drowsy. The record demonstrates a typical pattern of hypnagogic hypersynchrony – rhythmic, synchronous slow waves, in this case at a frequency of just over 5 Hz. This pattern is typically seen in infants and children, but sometimes appears as late as early adolescence.

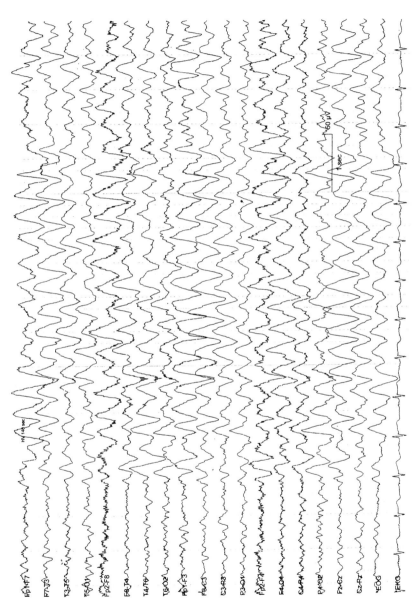

**A-19** Hyperventilation response. This recording in a 26-year-old woman demonstrates a normal response to hyperventilation. It consists of high-amplitude, synchronous, rhythmic delta waves with a bifrontal preponderance. Common in children, the response may persist well into adult life. The notation at the top of this example indicates that the burst occurred 140 seconds into hyperventilation.

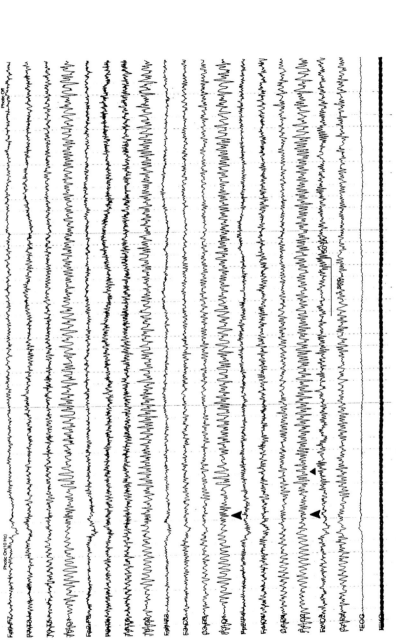

**A-20** Following (driving) response to photic stimulation. This example obtained during photic stimulation at 10 Hz evokes a following response (photic driving). Please note the alpha rhythm at 11.5 to 12 Hz in the first 2 seconds, followed by a 20-Hz rhythmic frequency at the start of the flash train (indicated by the arrow and the technician's note above). This in fact is a harmonic of the fundamental response (i.e. a response at 10 Hz). This may be appreciated after 2 seconds where the fundamental underlies the harmonic response.

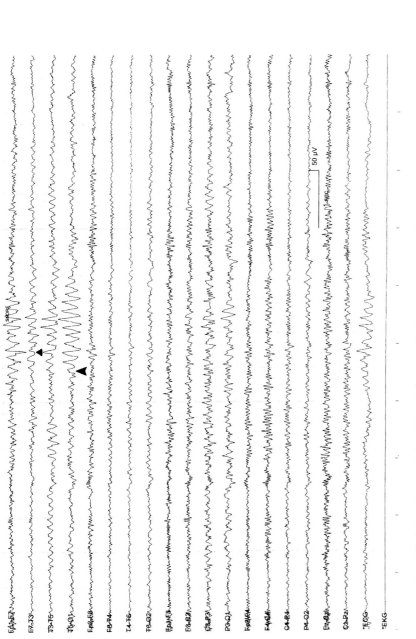

**A-21** Rhythmic mid-temporal theta. Formerly known as "psychomotor variant," rhythmic midtemporal theta, usually at 5 to 6 Hz, occurs mostly in young adults during early sleep stages. It consists of bursts of rhythmic sharply contoured theta activity (large arrow) lasting up to a few seconds. The bursts often occur independently on the two sides. This example from a drowsy young woman with syncopal attacks demonstrates the phenomenon with phase reversals at the left mid-temporal electrode (small arrow).

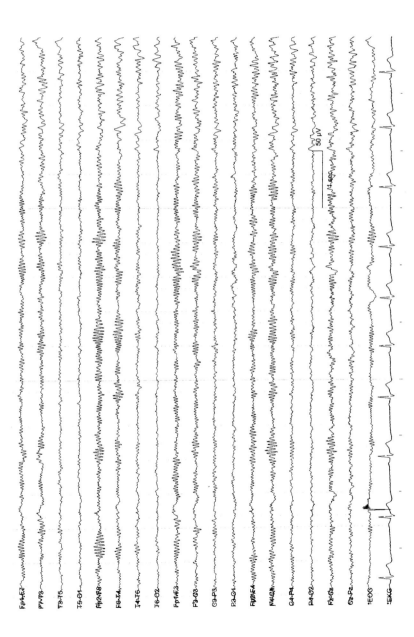

**A-22** Drug-induced beta activity. This record was obtained in an adult who was taking clonazepam. There is prominent drug-induced beta activity at 20 Hz, most prominent in the anterior head regions.

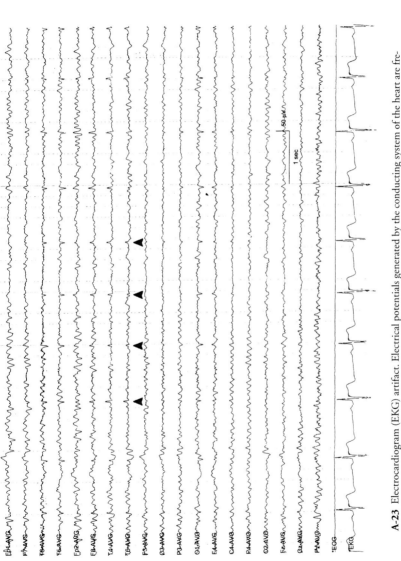

**A-23** Electrocardiogram (EKG) artifact. Electrical potentials generated by the conducting system of the heart are frequently reflected in the EEG and can produce an artifact that may be mistaken for intermittent sharp waves or spikes. In most laboratories a dedicated EKG channel makes identification relatively easy. This example demonstrates EKG artifact in multiple channels, coincident with the EKG recorded in the last channel. In some patients with higher voltage premature contractions, the artifact may occur intermittently, not rhythmically. In such instances the phase relationships are helpful in making a determination, but an EKG channel is indispensable. Note that EKG artifact is common in hypertensive and obese patients.

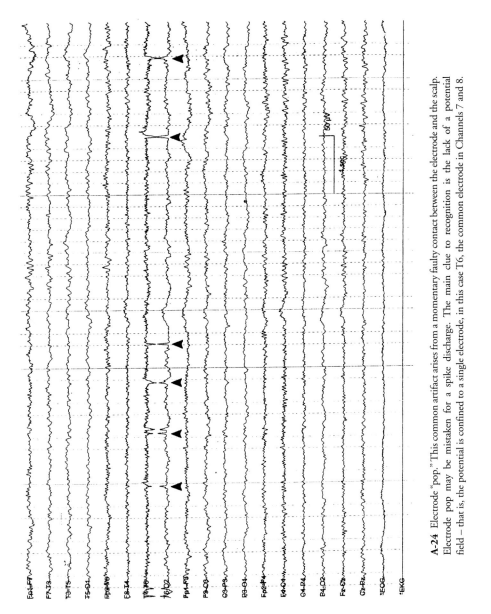

**A-24** Electrode "pop." This common artifact arises from a momentary faulty contact between the electrode and the scalp. Electrode pop may be mistaken for a spike discharge. The main clue to recognition is the lack of a potential field – that is, the potential is confined to a single electrode, in this case T6, the common electrode in Channels 7 and 8.

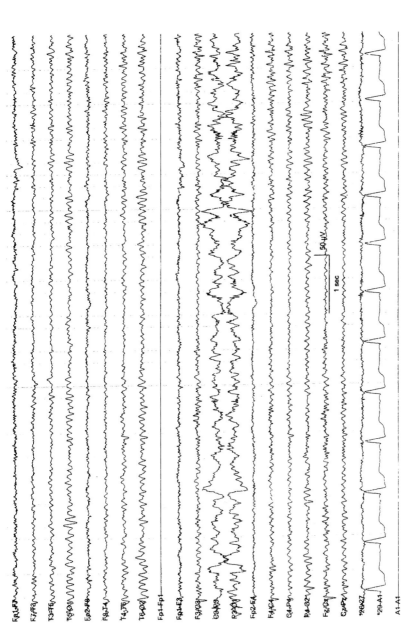

**A-25** Continual electrode artifact. This example demonstrates another electrode artifact due to the high impedance of the faulty electrode, in this case at P3, the common electrode. The artifact stands out from the normal cerebral activity in the remaining channels and demonstrates a typical mirror image appearance. Note that the technician should reapply the offending electrode soon after such an artifact appears!

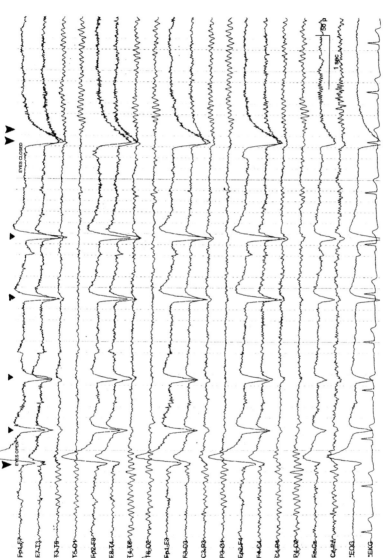

**A-26** Eye blink artifact. This example demonstrates eye-opening (large arrow) followed by eye blinks (small arrows) and eye closure (double arrow). Eye opening and closure artifact along with blinks are recorded mainly by the frontal electrodes. They are easily identified by their distribution, symmetry, and characteristic morphology. The high-voltage is due to the standing corneo-retinal potential (the cornea is positive with respect to the retina, measured in millivolts). The downward deflection results from the slight upward movement of the eye globe, the anteriorly placed electrodes (in input I of each channel) becoming momentarily positive with respect to channels in input II. Note that eye opening results in an upward deflection as the eye globe deviates downward and channels in input I one become relatively more negative with respect to input II.

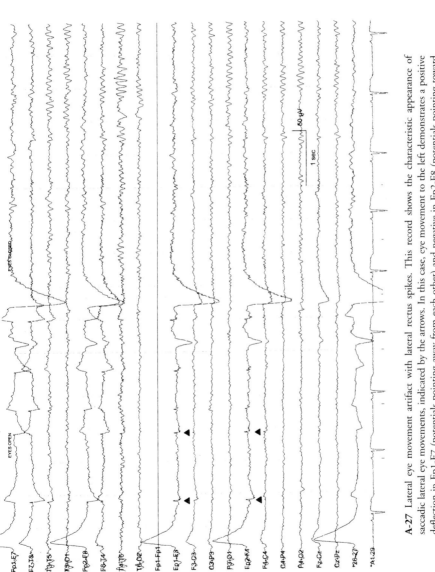

**A-27** Lateral eye movement artifact with lateral rectus spikes. This record shows the characteristic appearance of saccadic lateral eye movements, indicated by the arrows. In this case, eye movement to the left demonstrates a positive deflection in Fp1-F7 (potentials pointing away from each other) and negative in Fp2-F8 (potentials pointing toward each other – first large arrow). Movement to the right demonstrates the opposite (second large arrow). Horizontal nystagmus produces a similar artifact that is highly rhythmic. In channels Fp1-F3 and Fp2-F4, lateral rectus spikes are evident (small arrows).

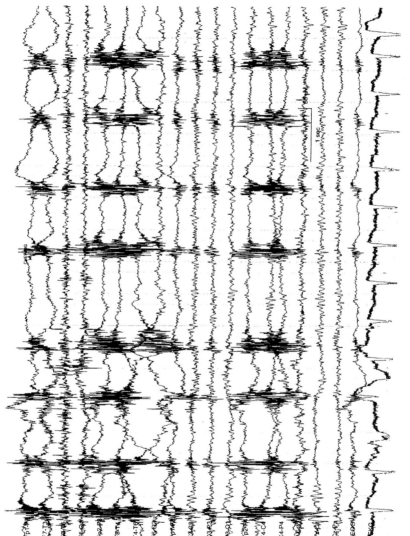

**A-28** Chewing artifact. In this example bursts of high-voltage muscle action potentials are due to the patient's chewing movements. Note the rhythmicity of the artifact, due to repetitive contraction of the masticatory muscles.

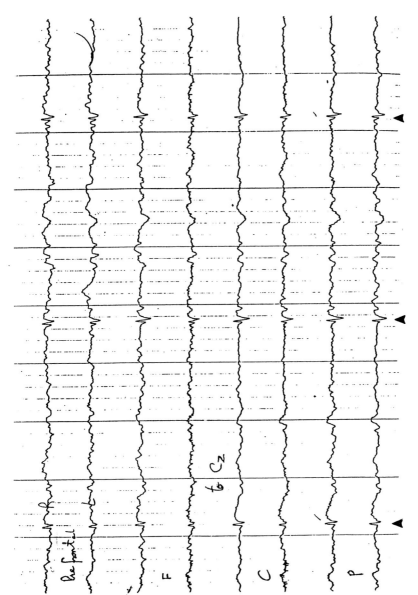

**A-29**  Intravenous (IV) drip artifact. This old paper recording demonstrates a relatively rare artifact occasionally seen in in-patient recordings. The spike-like discharges are presumably due to the electrically charged droplets as they descend in proximity to the recording electrodes. The clue to the non-physiological nature of the phenomenon is its precise periodicity. The technician should note the presence of the IV drip – this is a helpful bit of information.

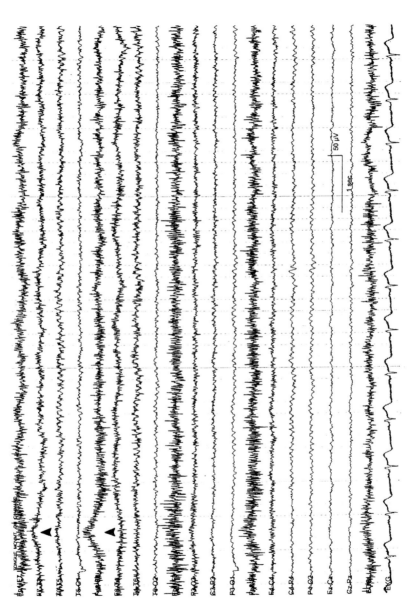

**A-30** Tongue movement artifact. This record contains continuous muscle activity in the anterior channels and low-amplitude delta waves, best seen in the frontotemporal channels. The slow waves are due to the subject's random tongue movements, indicated by the technician's remark at the top of the recording.

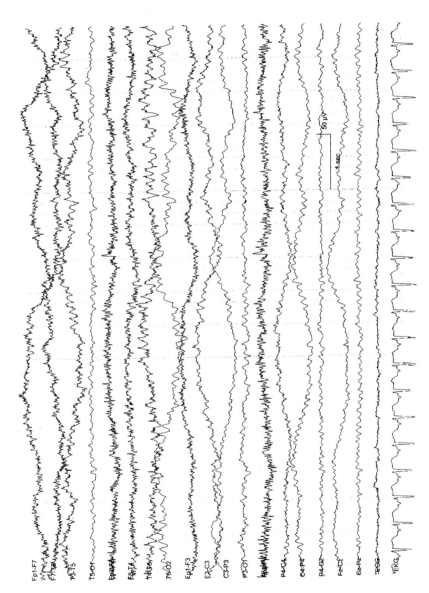

**A-31** Perspiration artifact. Perspiration produces an artifact that consists of very slow potentials, often with durations of several seconds. It produces an unstable baseline due to creation of a salt bridge with marked reduction of electrode impedance.

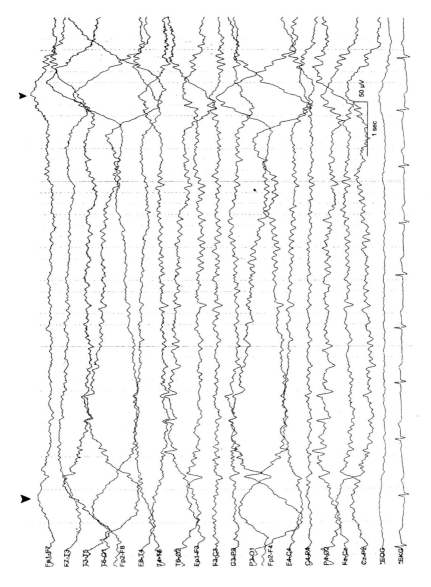

**A-32** Respirator artifact. This record was obtained from an intubated patient in an intensive care unit. The large-amplitude waves at either end of this strip correspond to the respirator setting. There was near-perfect periodicity throughout the tracing.

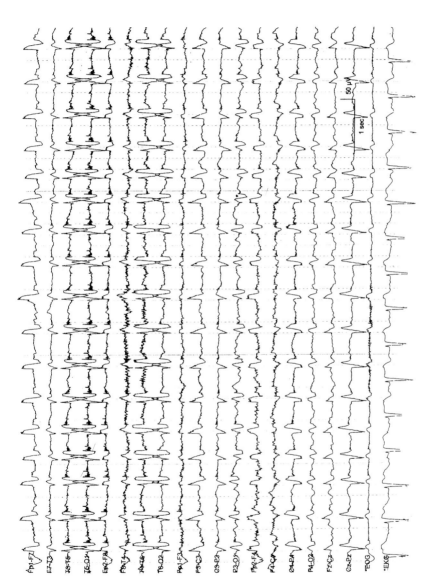

**A-33** Intraventricular assist device artifact. This impressive artifact was obtained from a comatose patient with an implanted intraventricular assist device. The waveform is of high-voltage and pervasive in all channels. Although the record is rendered uninterpretable, little cerebral activity can be made out during intervals between the artifacts.

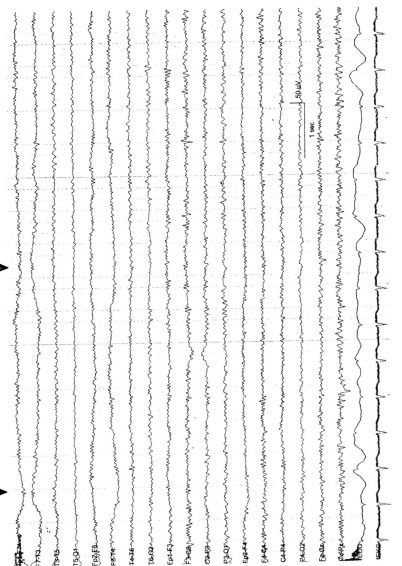

**A-34** Roving eye movements. This recording demonstrates an artifact produced by slow alternating lateral eye movements, shown as very slow waves in the frontotemporal channels. Note the alternating phase reversals. Such eye movements are often seen in early drowsiness.

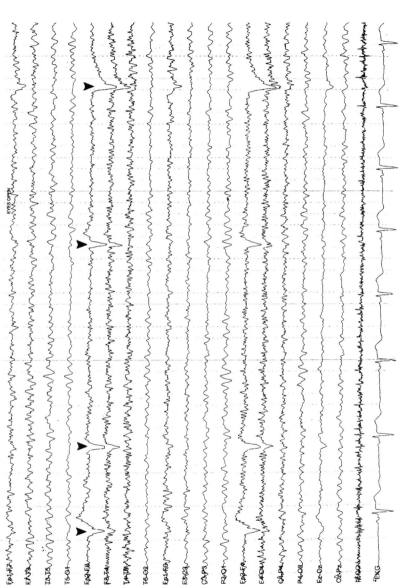

**A-35** Asymmetric eye blink artifact. The reader may be puzzled by this example where apparent typical eye blink artifacts appear only on the right side. The explanation is simple. The patient had a prosthetic left eye (thus, no corneo-retinal potential). Other causes of asymmetric eye movements include asymmetric electrode placement, skull defects, and extraocular muscle abnormalities.

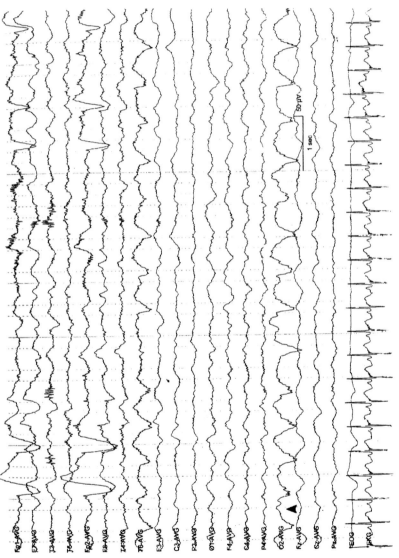

**A-36** Artifact due to a feeding pump. This is another example of a mechanical artifact. This is a 5-year-old boy in the pediatric intensive care unit. The high-amplitude rhythmic slow wave focus with maximal amplitude in the right occipital (O2) electrode was due to the circular motion of the feeding pump, situated close to the electrode wires. This turned out to be important, in that the pediatric neurologists, viewing the record without this information, felt the waves might represent epileptiform activity!

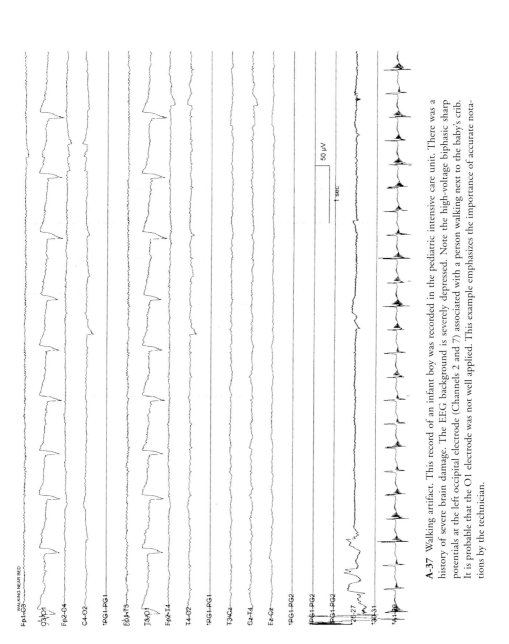

**A-37** Walking artifact. This record of an infant boy was recorded in the pediatric intensive care unit. There was a history of severe brain damage. The EEG background is severely depressed. Note the high-voltage biphasic sharp potentials at the left occipital electrode (Channels 2 and 7) associated with a person walking next to the baby's crib. It is probable that the O1 electrode was not well applied. This example emphasizes the importance of accurate notations by the technician.

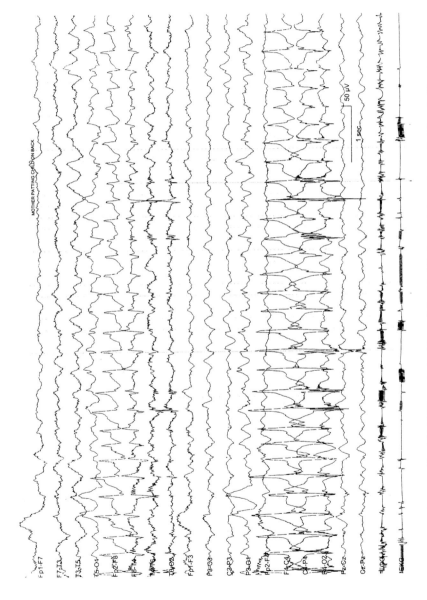

**A-38** Patting artifact. This EEG was obtained from a baby girl while she was sitting on her mother's lap. At this point her mother was patting her on the back. The high-voltage, rhythmic sharp potentials bear a superficial resemblance to a seizure discharge. There is, however, no understandable potential field. Again, the reader is aided by the technician's notation.

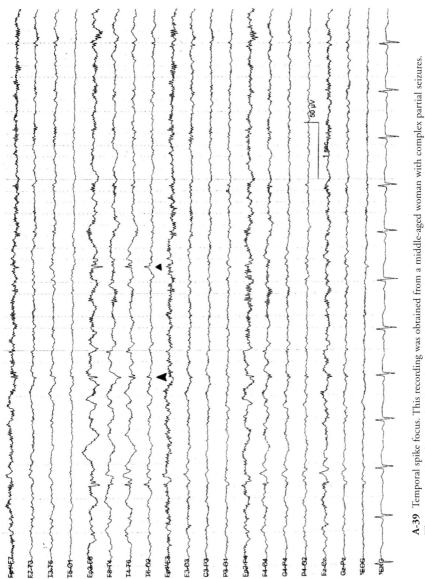

**A-39** Temporal spike focus. This recording was obtained from a middle-aged woman with complex partial seizures. There are repetitive, low-amplitude spikes with phase reversals at the right mid-temporal electrode (T4, large arrow), or between the anterior and mid temporal electrodes (F8–T4, small arrow).

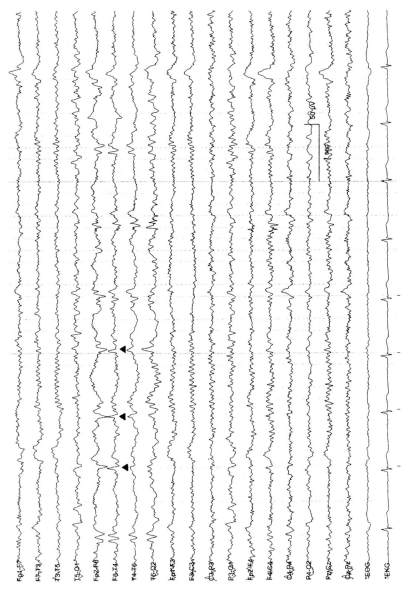

**A-40** Temporal spike focus. Another example of a spike focus in a patient with complex partial seizures. The spikes have a potential maximum at the right anterior temporal electrode (F8) and are followed by low-voltage slow waves. Note that the patient is asleep with fairly widely distributed 14 Hz sleep spindles.

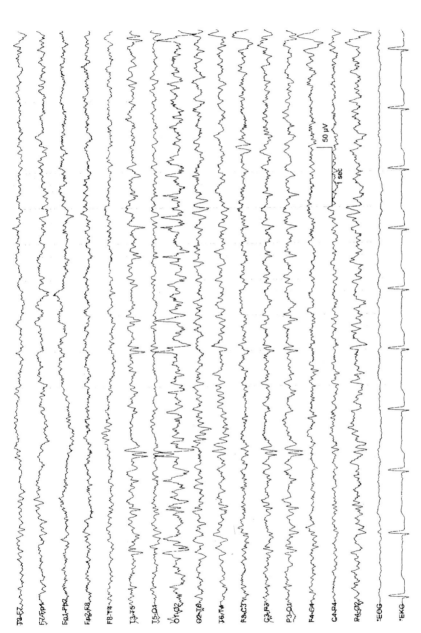

**A-41a** Occipital spike focus, bipolar recording. This is a record from a 32-year-old woman with a history of generalized tonic-clonic seizures. She never had associated visual symptoms and has been seizure-free for three years. In this circle or hat-band montage note the frequent high-voltage spikes with phase reversals between T5 and O1. Channel 7 does not reflect the spikes due to in-phase cancellation.

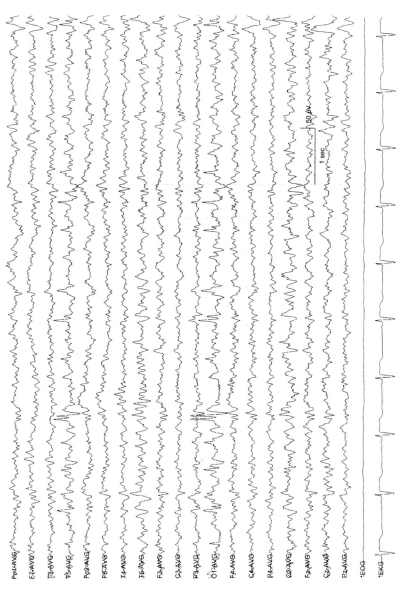

**A-41b** Occipital spike focus, referential recording. The same patient Atlas Figure A-41a, and same 10-second epoch of recording. Here, the spikes are evident in Channels 4 and 12 (T5 and O1). Note that the spike amplitude in these two channels is essentially identical. This leads to the in-phase cancellation referred to in the bipolar example.

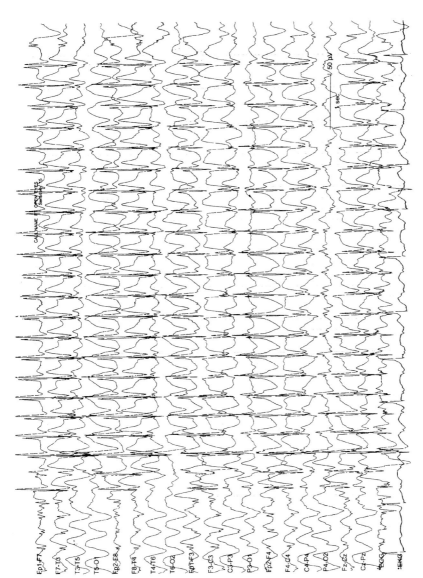

**A-42** Generalized typical spike-wave discharges in a child. This is a 6-year-old boy with absence epilepsy. An electrographic seizure was captured during hyperventilation. The record demonstrates a typical train of synchronous, high-voltage (up to 500 μV) 3 Hz spike-wave complexes. Note that at the top of the recording the technician called the patient's name and he opened his eyes, demonstrating some degree of responsivity.

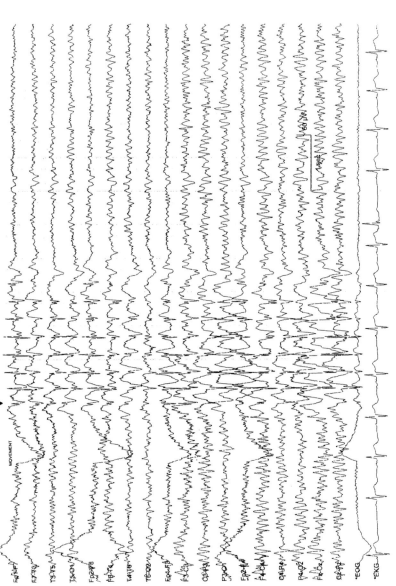

**A-43** Generalized spike-wave discharges in an adult. This record was taken from a 30-year-old man with a history of absence attacks in childhood with occasional generalized tonic–clonic seizures. He has had no major attacks for 20 years while taking valproate. He consulted his physician because of occasional slight lapses of attention. The record shows a 2-second train of generalized 3.5 Hz spike-wave complexes, followed by re-establishment of a well-developed alpha rhythm. Thus, this is an example of persistent primary generalized epilepsy in an adult.

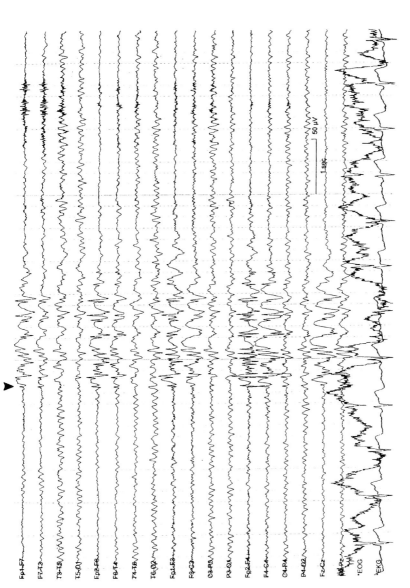

A-44  Generalized polyspike-wave discharges. This neurologically normal young woman has a history of generalized tonic-clonic seizures. Her record demonstrates bursts of polyspike-wave complexes with a bifrontal preponderance. In this example note the well-organized alpha preceding and following the 2.5-second burst. The patient likely has primary generalized epilepsy; although a frontal epilepsy with secondary generalization cannot definitely be ruled out.

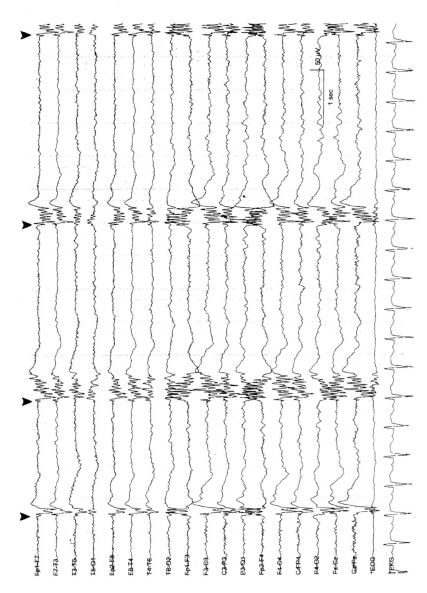

**A-45** Polyspikes. This is another example of polyspikes, recorded in a young man with generalized tonic-clonic seizures. Note the highly rhythmic spikes at 20 Hz, followed by a moderate amplitude delta wave. The discharges were activated during drowsiness.

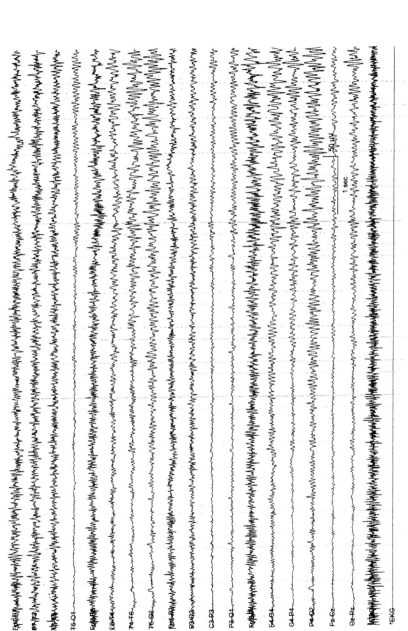

**A-46** Onset of a localization-related seizure. This recording in a 47-year-old woman with frequent complex partial seizures captures the onset of one of her events. Despite the muscle artifact in the frontal and left temporal regions, one can just make out a new, low-voltage 25 to 30 Hz rhythm in the right hemisphere during the first second of this plate (look at Channels 7, 8, and 14–16). The discharge gradually increases in amplitude and declines in frequency. The left hemisphere begins to participate during the seventh second (see Channels 4 and 12).

**A-47** Continuation of a localization-related seizure. This plate is a direct continuation of the previous example. Note the increase in amplitude of the discharge along with a pattern of polyrhythmicity – that is, admixed alpha and beta frequencies. There is an amplitude preponderance in the right posterior temporal region (Channels 7 and 8) and a wide distribution in the paracentral region (channels 13–16). There is now clear participation of the left hemisphere at lower voltage (compare with Atlas Figure A-46). During the event the patient's eyes were open and she was unresponsive. From this plate alone it would be difficult to identify the pattern as an electrographic seizure. This requires seeing the previously normal and symmetrical record as well as the onset of a new frequency in Figure A-46.

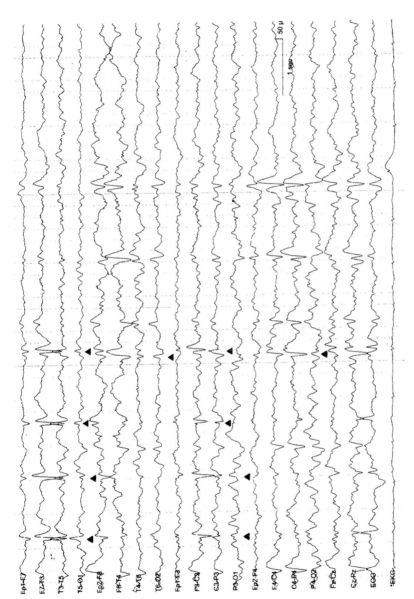

A-48  Centrotemporal spikes. This example was obtained from an 8-year-old boy with benign epilepsy of childhood with centrotemporal spikes (BECTS – formerly benign Rolandic epilepsy). The discharges recorded here are typical and consist of biphasic spikes appearing independently in the two hemispheres. Phase-reversals are noted at the mid temporal and central electrodes. Typically the spikes are activated by drowsiness as in this example. The alert reader will note an electrode artifact at F8 (Channels 5 and 6).

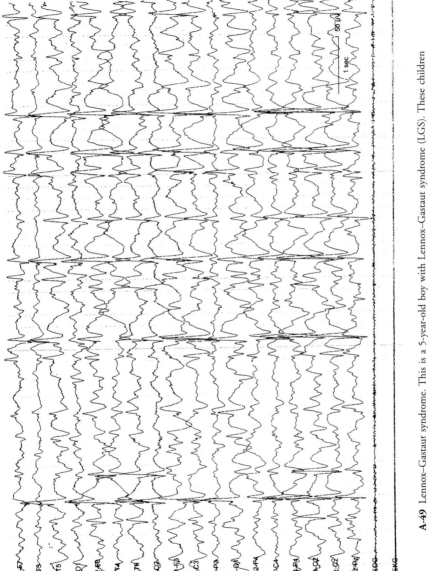

**A-49** Lennox–Gastaut syndrome. This is a 5-year-old boy with Lennox–Gastaut syndrome (LGS). These children suffer from multiple seizure types including atonic, myoclonic, generalized convulsive, and atypical absences. Mental retardation is usual. The EEG demonstrated generalized slow spike-wave discharges as in this example (compare with Atlas Figure A-42). Discharge amplitudes are high, in this case up to 600 μV (see calibration in lower right corner).

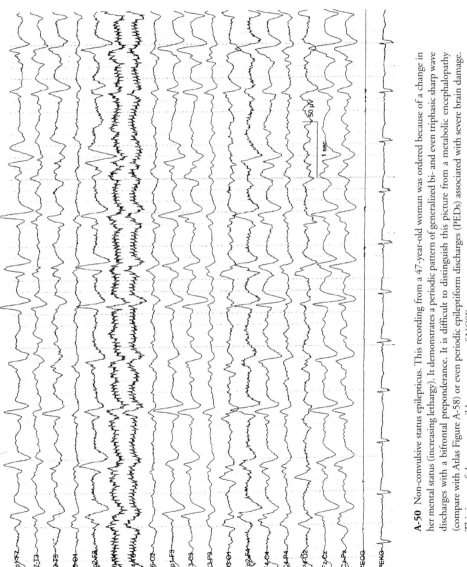

**A-50** Non-convulsive status epilepticus. This recording from a 47-year-old woman was ordered because of a change in her mental status (increasing lethargy). It demonstrates a periodic pattern of generalized bi- and even triphasic sharp wave discharges with a bifrontal preponderance. It is difficult to distinguish this picture from a metabolic encephalopathy (compare with Atlas Figure A-58) or even periodic epileptiform discharges (PEDs) associated with severe brain damage. This is one of the many possible appearances of NCSE.

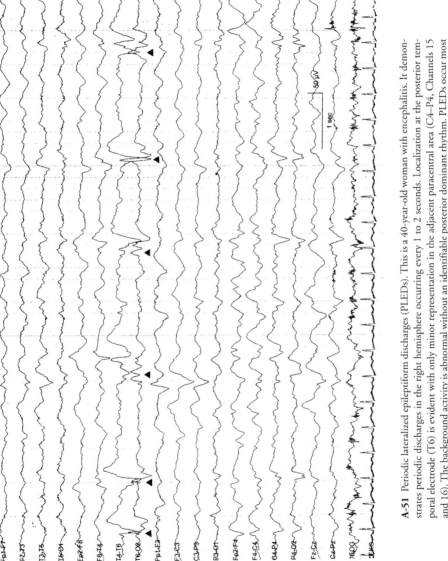

**A-51** Periodic lateralized epileptiform discharges (PLEDs). This is a 40-year-old woman with encephalitis. It demonstrates periodic discharges in the right hemisphere occurring every 1 to 2 seconds. Localization at the posterior temporal electrode (T6) is evident with only minor representation in the adjacent paracentral area (C4–P4, Channels 15 and 16). The background activity is abnormal without an identifiable posterior dominant rhythm. PLEDs occur most often in acute cerebral lesions such as stroke or encephalitis. They also may be associated with tumors.

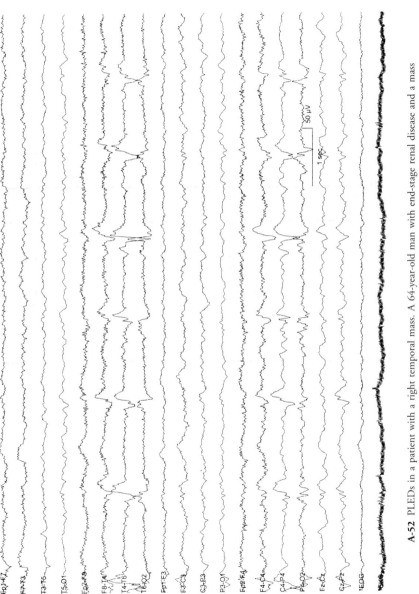

**A-52** PLEDs in a patient with a right temporal mass. A 64-year-old man with end-stage renal disease and a mass lesion in the right temporal lobe had a generalized convulsion five days before this EEG. Since that time he was noted to be somnolent. The record shows prominent periodic discharges in the right hemisphere with a repetition rate of about 1 per second. The background is diffusely slow without a posterior dominant rhythm.

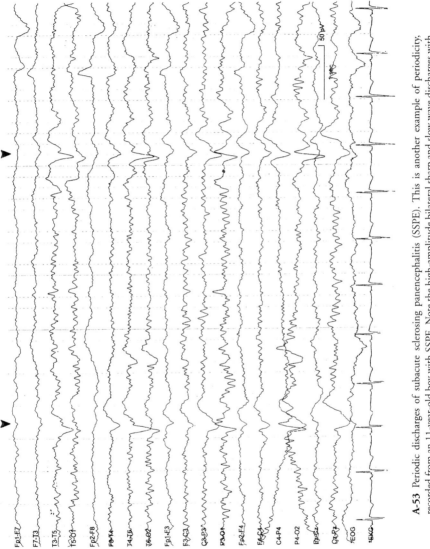

**A-53** Periodic discharges of subacute sclerosing panencephalitis (SSPE). This is another example of periodicity, recorded from an 11-year-old boy with SSPE. Note the high-amplitude bilateral sharp and slow wave discharges with a posterior preponderance, occurring at 6-second intervals. The discharges were associated with relatively slow myoclonic jerks.

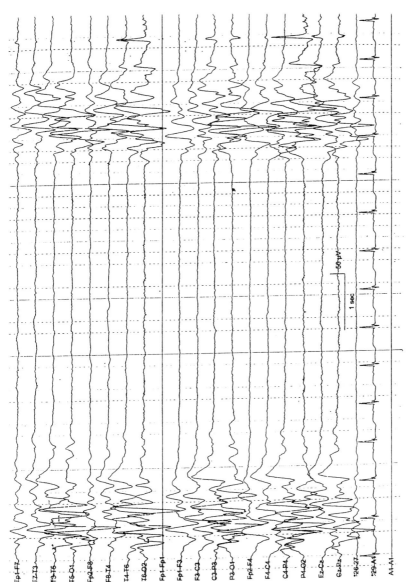

**A-54** Burst-suppression. This 76-year-old woman suffered a severe anoxic brain injury secondary to cardiogenic shock. Bursts of diffuse, irregular slow and sharp waves lasting about 1.5 seconds were noted throughout the tracing. Note the relative absence of background activity during interburst intervals. Burst-suppression, unless induced by general anesthesia, indicates severe cerebral injury, often due to an anoxic insult.

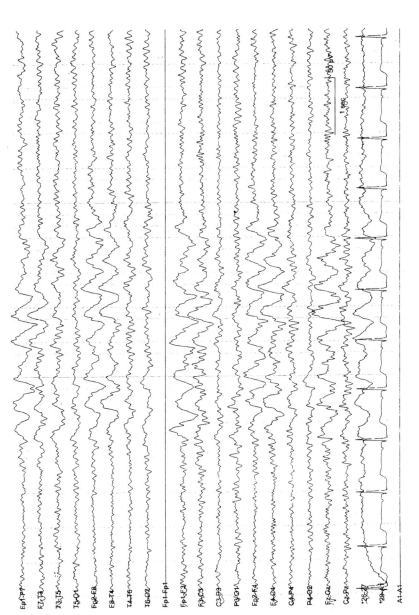

**A-55** Frontal intermittent rhythmic delta activity (FIRDA). This tracing was obtained in a 57-year-old woman with an intraventricular hemorrhage. Evident is a run of synchronous, rhythmic 2 Hz delta waves with a bifrontal preponderance. This EEG picture is typical of lesions involving deep midline structures, one of the causes being increased intracranial pressure. Deep tumors and even toxic-metabolic disorders may also produce FIRDA (see Atlas Figure A-56).

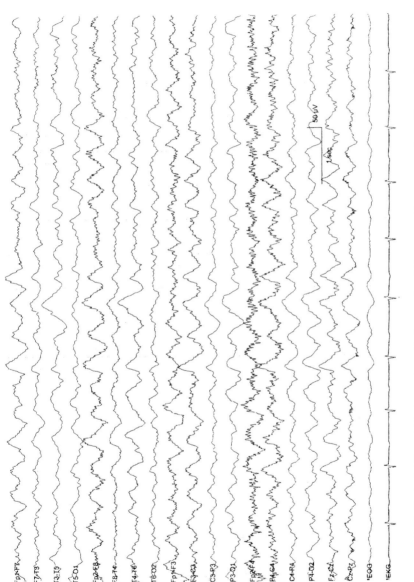

**A-56** Rhythmic bifrontal delta in a patient with drug overdose. This 29-year-old woman was admitted because of an overdose of Tylenol® and Percocet® . She was lethargic at the time of this EEG. The record is disorganized and shows rhythmic, symmetrical bifrontal delta activity at a frequency of 2 Hz.

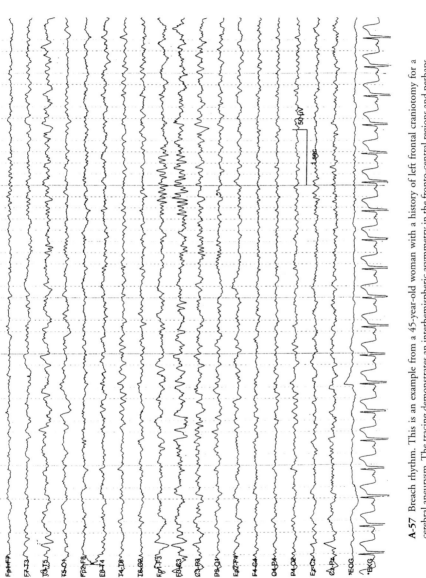

**A-57** Breach rhythm. This is an example from a 45-year-old woman with a history of left frontal craniotomy for a cerebral aneurysm. The tracing demonstrates an interhemispheric asymmetry in the fronto-central regions and perhaps slightly in the adjacent temporal area. There is increased background amplitude as well as slowing on the left side (Channels 9–11). Note the prominent sleep spindle on the left that is not represented on the right. This picture is secondary to the patient's skull defect along with some residual brain damage (breach = a broken or torn place or part: *Webster's New World College Dictionary*, 4th edition).

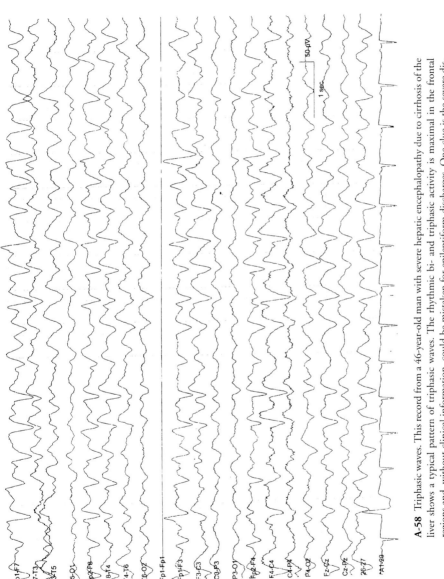

Fp1-F7
F7-T3
T3-T5
T5-O1
Fp2-F8
F8-T4
T4-T6
T6-O2

Fp1-Fp1
Fp1-F3
F3-C3
C3-P3
P3-O1
Fp2-F4
F4-C4
C4-P4
P4-O2
Fz-Cz
Cz-Pz
26-27
?A1+20

50 µV

1 sec.

**A-58** Triphasic waves. This record from a 46-year-old man with severe hepatic encephalopathy due to cirrhosis of the liver shows a typical pattern of triphasic waves. The rhythmic bi- and triphasic activity is maximal in the frontal regions and, without clinical information, could be mistaken for epileptiform discharges. One clue is the severe disruption of background activity, making a metabolic encephalopathy more likely. Triphasic waves, most often associated with hepatic encephalopathy, may be seen in other metabolic encephalopathies, for example in a setting of renal failure.

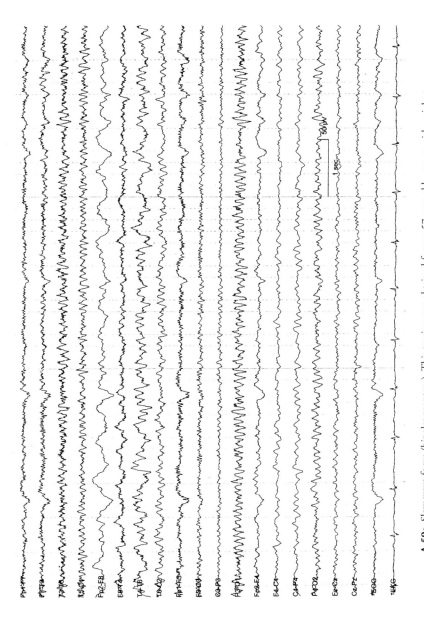

**A-59a** Slow wave focus (bipolar montage). This tracing was obtained from a 57-year-old woman with a right temporal astrocytoma. Note the continual moderate amplitude delta waves in the left temporal region with phase reversals between the anterior and mid-temporal electrodes (Channels 5–7). The background rhythmic activity is disrupted, and minimal representation of the slowing is present in the adjacent paracentral region.

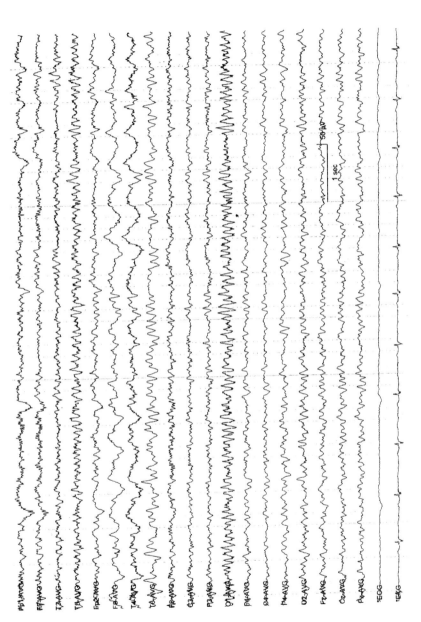

**A-59b** Slow wave focus (common average reference montage). This is the same EEG segment as Atlas Figure A-62, but displayed in common average reference recording. Note the maximum amplitude of the delta activity in common average reference recording. This indicates that the focus is between these two electrodes. Remember: with referential recording (Channels 5 and 6). This indicates that the focus is between these two electrodes. Remember: with referential recording the localizing principle is amplitude, whereas, in bipolar recording, localization is conveyed by the phase reversal.

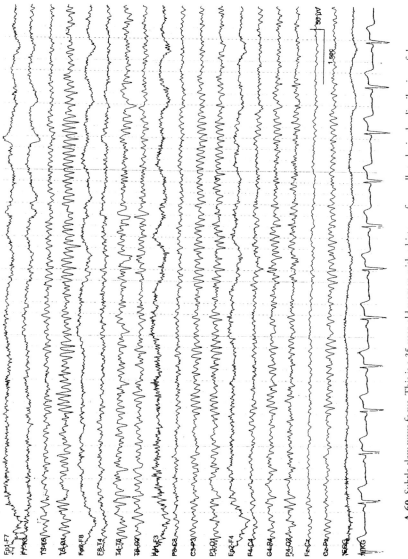

**A-60** Subtle slow wave focus. This is a 35-year-old woman with a history of a small stroke in the distribution of the right middle cerebral artery. This is an example of subtler focal slowing than seen in Atlas Figure A-59a. Note intermittent theta activity at T6 (Channels 7 and 8) along with disruption of the alpha.

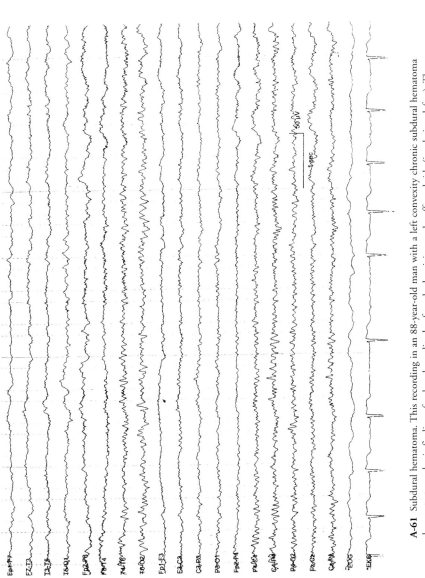

**A-61** Subdural hematoma. This recording in an 88-year-old man with a left convexity chronic subdural hematoma demonstrates a classic finding of reduced amplitude of cerebral activity on the affected side (insulation defect). There is also disruption of background activity. It is difficult to decide, based on this page, whether there is any associated slowing.

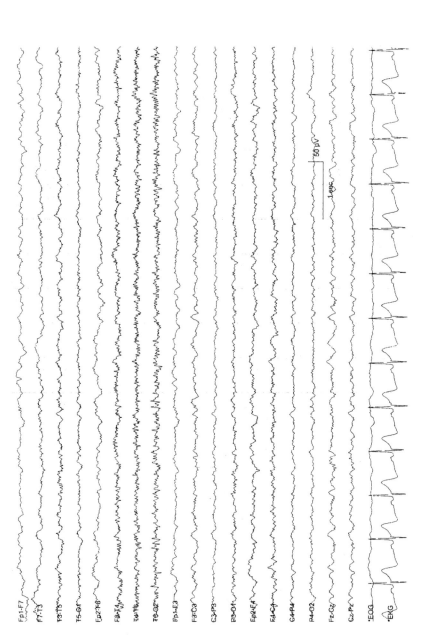

**A-62** Dementia. This record was obtained in a 67-year-old man with dementia, probably Alzheimer's disease. Note the lack of organized background rhythmic activity. There is generalized, relatively low-voltage slowing in both theta and delta ranges. No focal or lateralized features are evident.

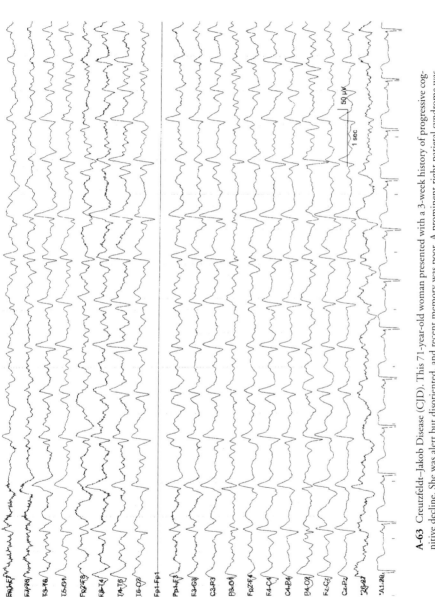

**A-63** Creutzfeldt–Jakob Disease (CJD). This 71-year-old woman presented with a 3-week history of progressive cognitive decline. She was alert but disoriented, and recent memory was poor. A prominent right parietal syndrome was evident, including left-sided neglect. Also observed was intermittent rhythmic jerking of the left arm. The record demonstrates synchronous periodic sharp wave discharges occurring every 800 to 1000 ms. Note the potential maximum in the posterior quadrants. The patient did not have a brain biopsy, but the Flair MRI demonstrated findings were consistent with CJD.

# INDEX

Page numbers in *italics* refer to illustrations.